Nursing At Its Finest

Deanna Mackey, RN

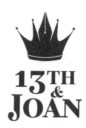

13TH & JOAN

For permission requests, write to the publisher, addressed "Attention: Permissions Coordinator," 205 N. Michigan Avenue, Suite #810, Chicago, IL 60601. 13th & Joan books may be purchased for educational, business or sales promotional use. For information, please email the Sales Department at sales@13thandjoan.com.

Printed in the U. S. A.

First Printing, December 2020.

Library of Congress Cataloging-in-Publication Data has been applied for.

ISBN: 978-1-953156-27-3

For my daughter, Zamora, who inspires me to be
a better role model every day.

For my mom, Tina, who molded me into the persistent,
hard working, compassionate individual that I am today.

To my sister, Detra, who supported me in ways
that no one else could.

To all of the frontline workers, especially my fellow nurses,
during this unfortunate time.

We SEE you and we THANK you.

Dreams are lovely. But they are just dreams. Fleeting, ephemeral, pretty. But dreams do not come true just because you dream them. It's hard work that makes things happen. It's hard work that creates change.

—Shonda Rhimes

Deanna Mackey, has written a must read book for anyone considering nursing as a career choice. In this book, she shares her insight and wisdom on the complexities of life and nursing in general. This book is a wonderful way to welcome novice nurses on their journey towards professional self development, confidence and compassion. Life lessons learned: never give up, follow your dreams, fight for what you believe in, you too and will become a great Nurse just like myself and friend Deanna. I wish I had this book to guide me along the way in my college years, as I took many different paths to achieve yet the same goal, which was to become a Registered Nurse.

—Shardae Crawley, BSN, RN

"In this impressive debut, Deanna Mackey outlines the apprehensions of a nurse or a nursing student . This is a great playbook for a successful journey in nursing!"

—Tiombi Jackson, BSN, RN

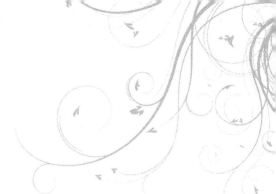

"Deanna Mackey was able to touch both the new nurse and the seasoned nurse. This book gives insight to the new nurses beginning their journey into the nursing world and provides nostalgic memories for the seasoned nurse.

A great read that masters the ability to make the writer's personal journey into the world of nursing so relatable to both the rookie nurse and the veteran nurse, describing the rollercoaster of emotions to expect throughout the ride."

—Mineisha Green, BSN, RN

"Energetic, Knowledgeable, Articulate, Detail-Oriented, Passionate, Exuberant, and Dedicated to the field of Nursing. There is no other way to describe Deanna Mackey, Registered Nurse. She has displayed these characteristics without fail from the first day we met working together. The numerous compliments from those she has helped says it all. Sit down, relax, and get ready to enjoy her invaluable erudition."

—Marcus Nicholson, MBA, MSN, RN

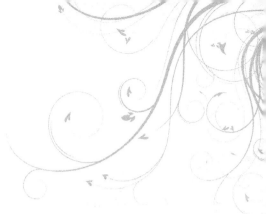

Contents

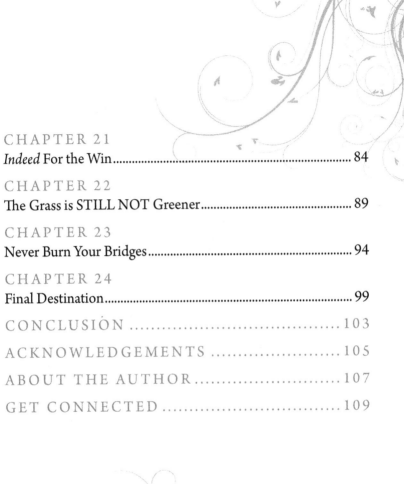

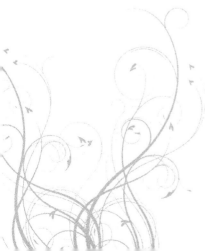

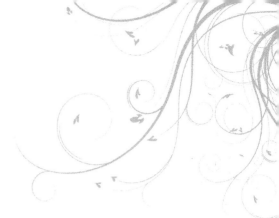

Preface

I started writing this book while working in my last hospital position as a registered nurse and after speaking with a close friend of mine who is also a nurse. We work in different states but experienced mostly the same scenarios while working, and that inspired us to tell our stories.

I felt that I had a story to tell that could influence others that were following the same path as me. I wanted to create a self-help/autobiography that would assist others. If I could influence an upcoming nurse, be relatable to a nurse already in the field, or simply get the attention of a layperson interested in knowing more about this field, that would mean my book served its purpose.

I think the route that I took to become a nurse makes me unique because I had to overcome some obstacles that not everyone has to overcome. Also, coming straight into the nursing field working on a psychiatric/behavioral health unit as a new nurse is a challenge in itself.

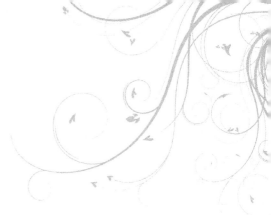

Introduction

As children, we are always asked what we want to be when we grow up. It's one of those aspects of our life that our parents/guardians, role models, and teachers want us to prepare for. Sometimes children know exactly what they want to be and sometimes they don't. Sometimes what we say we are going to be, we end up being in a completely different field. Our life experiences and upbringings mold us into who we are meant to be.

For me, I knew immediately what I wanted to be when I grew up. Becoming a registered nurse was always a life goal of mine, and I knew that there was no other career field I'd rather be in. Through all the adversity and challenges that I faced, I never let anything hold me back from achieving that goal.

For the past seven years of being a nurse, I have seen and experienced a plethora of events. I've tested the waters by working in several different areas of nursing, including psychiatric/behavioral health nursing. Every position has made me question if this was the best career choice for me. Was this truly my calling or was I misjudging it all? I thought that once I graduated nursing school and received my nursing license that my career would flourish and I would finally be in a position that I could truly fall in love with. I didn't want just a J-O-B, I'd already had several of those;

I wanted a career that I loved. I didn't want it to feel like work; I wanted it to feel as though I was fulfilled.

I had never felt that feeling, no matter how hard I tried to get there or what experience I was getting. Although I had been thankful for every opportunity, I still was on the search for *my* dream job. Once I finally found it, I took a moment to truly digest all that I had been through with each and every nursing job that I had possessed.

Reminiscing about all those opportunities and everything that came with them—the positives, heartaches, blood, sweat and tears—brought me to writing this book. I wanted to be able to share my story because I felt like it was worth listening to. I felt that I needed to allow others to be that fly on the wall that wants to see and hear everything without actually being seen.

If you're questioning a career path in nursing, are already a nurse, or just want more insight on this challenging yet rewarding job, this will surely give you some answers. This isn't *every* nurse's experience, but it is a guide on what to expect and how you can get there. I hope that this book will inspire each and every one of you.

A Little Girl With a Dream

*E*ver since I was a little girl, I knew that working in the medical field was my calling. Watching the show "Trauma: Life in the E.R." on TLC with my dad, as well as other medical shows, allowed me to gain a deeper interest in the medical field. At first, I wanted to become a doctor, but after learning and seeing the role of a nurse, I knew nursing would be my true calling. Nurses are the backbone of healthcare; they know what the person is going through before the doctor, they spend the most time with their patients, they are that patient's shoulder to cry on and their hand to hold. I knew that I possessed all of these qualities as an individual and that this truly was my calling.

Once I knew what I wanted to be when I grew up, I took every opportunity to stay on that path. I volunteered at the local hospital as a "Volunteen" in high school to gain more experience, while also obtaining my required community service hours. I was accepted into the Academy of Medical Careers at my high school in my junior year. I was also accepted into the Acceleration Program for health and science majors at my first college, Virginia Commonwealth University (VCU). All of these opportunities assisted in my learning of what the medical field entailed and gave me the knowledge I needed to gain about the human body. With that said, I knew that I was ready to apply to nursing school.

During the summer of 2007, while in the Acceleration Program, I met one of my best friends today, Shardae. I found out that she wanted to be a nurse also, and we have been friends ever since. She thought I was mean at first, but once we started getting to know each other, she knew she couldn't live without me.

At the end of our first semester, we both applied to the nursing program and were anxious to get our acceptance letters in the mail. We both were starting to take our prerequisites and had above a 3.0, so we just knew that we'd get in. Mid-January had approached, and we knew our letters would soon come in the mail. She received her letter and told me her response first. Unfortunately, she received the infamous "We regret to inform you that you have not been selected." I could hear the disbelief and sadness in her tone, and that only made me extremely nervous to open my letter. As I was opening up my letter, I was praying to God I get to read those promising words, while squeezing my eyes closed. As I unfolded the letter and opened my eyes, I was reading the first line, which read, "You have been waitlisted." I didn't know how to feel. I was mad that I wasn't accepted but also slightly happy that they wanted me enough to waitlist me. I knew that I at least had a small chance of getting in if someone couldn't afford it, someone decided not to attend, or if someone dropped out or didn't meet their requirements in time for the start of the program. Whether or not any of that happened, I knew that nursing was my passion, and I couldn't see myself doing anything else in life. Giving up wasn't an option, so I would continue taking my prerequisites.

We all know the basic classes every nursing program requires the applicant to take: biology, chemistry, Psychology 101, sociology, microbiology, nutrition, pathophysiology.... sound familiar??

Oh, and how could I forget the dreadful anatomy and physiology? Thankfully, I didn't have to take Anatomy I and II and Physiology I and II, like some programs offer. The anatomy lecture and lab that I took was one full semester as well as physiology the following semester. But of course, without passing anatomy, you couldn't take physiology the following semester. So during my first semester of my sophomore year, I was taking anatomy, which is already challenging in itself. During this time, I had a bad break-up, and I allowed it to cloud my studying. After that one failed lab exam, I learned very quickly that I'd better strap up and get it together. I came to college for one thing only, and that was to get that nursing degree. From then on, I made sure to continue to do well and never let anything or anyone get in my way.

I planned on only applying once more to VCU's nursing program by the spring of my sophomore year, since I never was picked from the waitlist. Once again, I waited for my letter to come in the mail. Unfortunately, I was waitlisted again. I really became discouraged at this point because I began to think maybe I wasn't doing enough or good enough to be accepted. I had above a 3.0 GPA, and even continued to volunteer at VCU's Child Development Center after my 20-hour class requirement was met. I truly loved working with the toddlers. Since I wanted to possibly become a labor & delivery nurse in the future, I figured this would be a great opportunity to have. I had great references also, so at this point I didn't know what to do. I called the nursing program to ask them what they are looking for when they reviewed the applications. I learned that they didn't even go through all of the applications and dispute who to choose because they received so many applications. They would literally go through so many—let's say 200 as an example—and choose their 20 students for the upcoming class. After that they either waitlist or deny your application. It's definitely first come first serve, amongst other things.

I then had to look at my options and make the best decision for my situation. I was already paying over $30,000 a year to attend VCU, being an out-of-state student. Of course, the majority of that was paid through financial aid and other grants and scholarships I had applied for and received separately. However, I was still paying over $5,000 out of pocket per semester to attend, which meant this young lady worked her butt off to continue to attend VCU. That also meant I needed a plan B if I wanted to graduate on time without paying any more money than I had to. At one point, after discussing this with my mom and sister, they suggested I transfer to an in-state college. However, I refused; I was going to do everything in my power to stay and graduate at VCU. The summer of my sophomore year, I even applied and got accepted into a summer program for health and science majors called HERO. Every student was assigned a mentor, and you had to work in their lab and carry out the research that they were currently working on. Very interesting research, plus I got paid for it of course.

Prior to my junior year, I met with my advisor, who suggested an equivalent major I could change to. This would still allow me to graduate on time as planned. That major would be psychology. All of the classes I had taken up until that point would still amount to the same credits and classes allowed under that psychology curriculum.

As my senior year approached, I knew that I had to start looking at nursing programs again. I had already completed just about all of the general prerequisites required by most nursing programs, so I knew that I would be able to go straight into my core nursing classes. However, I still had to make sure my credits would transfer and would be acceptable to whatever program I was accepted into. I had researched second degree nursing programs, which are basically programs for students who have a bachelor's degree in something other than nursing. This would be perfect for me, and it was only another two years. After searching multiple programs, I ended up applying to Bowie State University (BSU), Salisbury University (SU), and VCU once again. I did want to apply to the University of Maryland, but I had to take that lovely Test of Essential Academic Skills (TEAS) test. I didn't pass, so that choice was out.

Applying to these nursing programs also meant I had to apply to the actual universities and get accepted before the nursing programs would accept me. While I awaited my acceptance letters, I still had to finish off strong with my current degree. It was time to "apply to graduate" during the winter break of my senior year (2010). It was the week before the spring semester would start, and I had already registered for my classes prior to the winter break. As I was going through the application, I realized that one of the requirements included having at least 45 credits in upper level courses. Unfortunately, unbeknownst to me, I was 11 credits shy from meeting that requirement.

I knew I had to think of a plan fast. I still needed to take two of the classes I had registered for as prerequisites for the nursing programs I had applied to. Those classes were Chemistry 101 with the lab and microbiology with the lab. Because these weren't three or four credit classes, I had to replace those with classes that were, while still making sure I maintained my requirements for my psychology degree. Since the semester was about to start, there were slim to no classes left to choose from. Luckily, I found enough to suffice the graduate requirement. Most of them were criminal justice courses.

I was now registered for 18 credits for the spring semester at VCU. However, I still needed to find somewhere to take chemistry and microbiology. Luckily, after further research, I found an independent study option at Mountain State University (MSU) that had those classes. After registering, I had to make sure my current college, VCU, would allow me to do so. Thankfully, I was cleared and was now taking 26 credit hours total, on top of working 20 hours a week. I didn't know how I'd get through these next four and half months, but I knew half-assing it was not an option.

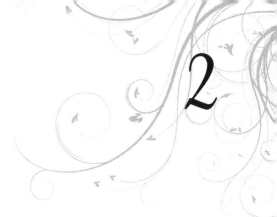

2

The Decision

While I busted my ass with these 26 credits, I waited on my acceptance letters to the nursing schools I had applied to. If I can recall correctly, BSU's letter came first. Although I called and specifically asked questions about my application prior to applying and knew that I met all of their requirements, they sent me a letter stating my application was incomplete. I knew that this was false and contested it. It was an error on their part, and they later corrected it and accepted my application. However, due to minor errors as such and doing a bit more research on their school and nursing program, I decided that wasn't the school for me.

Next was VCU's letter, which once again stated that I was placed on the waiting list. I didn't allow myself to get upset because I expected that outcome based on the last two times that I had applied. I did let my manager at the time know about it. Since he worked for VCU and knew someone that worked for the School of Nursing, he offered to put in a word for me. I agreed, although I was having second thoughts due to the costs, demanding class schedule, and the fact that I've always been one to truly earn what I've worked for. I knew if VCU decided to accept me, that it was only because of my manager putting a good word in for me. However, if I had no other options, I at least wanted something to fall back on.

I then got my acceptance letter from SU. I knew that I had already gotten accepted into their university, so I was praying that this letter was an acceptance letter into their nursing program. As I opened the letter, I was very anxious and nervous about what to expect. I pulled the letter out and there it was: the moment of truth. I glanced down at the letter, and it read, "Congratulations Ms. Mackey, you have been accepted into our nursing program." I smiled from ear to ear because I knew that I had finally got the opportunity that I had been waiting on for so long; I knew that I was one step closer to fulfilling my childhood dream.

Salisbury's nursing program was only three semesters, which included winter and summer breaks. It would be in my home state, so that meant no more out-of-state tuition. Although it wasn't located in the most desirable location, I knew that I had one purpose: to do my work, pass my classes, and graduate. Nothing else was important. I had already lived and experienced the "college life" at VCU. Plus, I'd only be there for one and a half years, which would fly by. I couldn't wait to respond with my decision. Being that this was a second-degree program, I most definitely needed to keep doing well while I finished out my last semester at VCU. The main requirement to be in that program was to have a bachelor's degree. Luckily, being the studious individual that I was raised to be, I graduated with honors, cum laude. I was so proud of myself, given the challenges I had faced that semester, taking 26 credit hours, and still having a life. I DID THAT!!

The icing on the cake was that I did in fact end up getting accepted into VCU's nursing program. About two weeks before graduation, I got an email from VCU's School of Nursing saying that I was accepted. They were literally giving me a few days to make a decision and turn in a $200 deposit. I thanked God for Salisbury seeing my potential and accepting me through a mere application and recommendation letters. As compared to VCU, a school I'd attended for four years with my GPA always being A/B average, where I'd volunteered and worked and received scholarships, and they never truly saw my potential. Had my manager never spoken up for me, they never would've accepted me as last minute as they did. Plus, I knew I couldn't afford to continue to attend VCU. It was time for my next step in this journey to be a registered nurse.

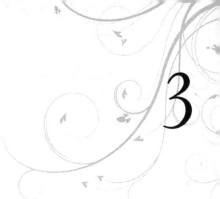

3

Post Grad I

That journey couldn't start until I took one more prerequisite required for SU's nursing program. That prerequisite was pathophysiology. I had no choice but to once again find an online course. Thankfully, I was able to find one that would be accepted. I took that course at the beginning of my summer break while I worked.

I was blessed to get a job with my psychology degree working as a social service designee at a nursing home. That's just a fancy name for a social worker's assistant. I was so thankful for that job because I not only got paid well, but I also was able to see firsthand what my future might consist of. It also allowed me to understand from a social worker's perspective how the healthcare system worked.

My position consisted of interviewing new admission residents, re-admitting residents, and the long-term residents. The questions consisted of their medical history, mental health, and memory questions. Most importantly, I interacted a lot with the other staff, including the nurses, CNAs/GNAs, director of the facility, and the physicians. The ones that I grew close to, including my manager, knew how much I dreamed of becoming a nurse, and they were very welcoming in allowing me to experience as much as possible on the job. Although that experience was very beneficial and rewarding for me, I knew that I didn't necessarily want to be a nurse in a nursing home. By simply witnessing the nurse to patient ratio, as well as how short staffed it seemed to be, and the population of the residents, I knew that the nursing home environment wasn't for me. I knew I preferably wanted to care for infants/children, but if not, then a range of adult ages.

Although I completed all of the prerequisites necessary to attend SU's nursing program that fall, I still had to pay off the money owed for taking those extra courses at MSU. I had to pay that off in order to get my transcript from them to turn into SU before the deadline. Luckily, with the rate of pay I was getting at the nursing home and me getting that job just in time, I was able to pay my bill off just in time. I truly believe everything happens for a reason, and He is always on time. As hard as I worked and as stressed out I had been going through all of this, it was all worth it because I was able to meet my goal and attend SU's nursing program in the fall of 2011. I not only received enough financial aid to attend, but I also received the Robert Wood Johnson Foundation New Careers in Nursing Scholarship, a $10,000 scholarship. I was so thankful for that scholarship because I was able to eliminate some of the loan money I had received.

4

Nursing School Begins

August of 2011 was the start of my nursing program. That first semester of nursing school consisted of four classes: Med-Surg Part 1 with the clinical, Health Assessment, and the Introduction to Professional Nursing Practice. This first semester, from the very beginning was a rude awakening for me. I was so used to not having to study as hard throughout all the years I had been in school, including the courses I took at VCU, while still getting at least a B. I actually studied for the first exam and received a C. I knew then that nursing school was totally different than what I was used to. I would definitely need to put in the work if I wanted to pass. That meant better time management, asking as many questions as possible, actually going to the library, and studying with my peers.

The first day of clinicals was exciting yet overwhelming, once our assignment was given to us. My clinicals took place on the orthopedic floor of the local hospital. Our clinical instructor was very welcoming but also quite critical of us. We of course had to get as much information as possible from our assigned patient and their clinical history from the computer and/or paper chart in order to complete our dreaded 50-page long care plan. I may be exaggerating slightly, but all those that can relate know exactly what I'm talking about.

She had us partner up in twos, and we had one assigned patient to care for on our 8-hour shift. My classmate and I had an older woman who'd had hip surgery two days prior. We were basically her nurses for the day. So we were responsible for administering her ordered medications, making and changing her bed sheets if needed, assisting her with using the bathroom, and any other necessary duties for the day. While doing this, we needed to ask her as many questions as possible to get her subjective perspective of being in the hospital as well as clinical information that was in her paper chart and electronic chart.

At some point, the patient rang her call bell, so we both went in to see what she needed. She said she had to use the bathroom, and since she'd just had hip surgery, it wasn't safe for her to get out of bed. So of course, we had to put the fracture bed pan underneath her while she lay in bed. This was a struggle in itself since those darn things are always confusing on which direction it is supposed to go. Then when you finally realize the correct way it should go, the patient has already used the bathroom and the urine is all over the bedsheets. Anyway, in a matter of minutes, she was finished. She had a bowel movement and I will never forget how queasy the smell of it made me. Fortunately, the patient didn't see my face, but my classmate did, and she suggested I just go ahead and dump the bedpan while she finished cleaning her up. She was a small lady, so my classmate was able to hold her on her own. I literally almost vomited when I took that bedpan into the bathroom. I knew then that that was my weakness. Just like some people, even nurses, can't stand the sight of blood or some other bodily fluid, the sight and odor of a bowel movement is definitely not my cup of tea.

As the day went on, we gathered as much information as possible in order to complete our assignment that night. Before we left for the day, our instructor went over what was expected from us on this assignment. I always dreaded doing care plans and never understood why they were so long because I just didn't foresee having to do all of this when I finally became a nurse. That didn't matter because I knew I'd be doing these for another year. I had a lot of mistakes and things that I could've added or explained more. For instance, for all the medications she was ordered, we needed to know their action, side effects, and the specific reason as to why that patient was taking them. We also had to know all of their lab work and why that particular patient's labs might've been abnormal based on their condition. Each clinical allowed me to gain a better understanding of what I needed to be paying attention to during that clinical day and particularly that patient.

While trying to keep it together through nursing school, my older sister was getting married that December, and of course, I was the maid of honor. Honestly, I was still a struggling college student, so my money was limited. However, I still tried to enjoy myself when I had free time and do as much as I could to help plan and coordinate my sister's wedding festivities. I also wished I could've made her bridal shower and definitely her bachelorette weekend more memorable, but I knew that she was thankful for what I was able to do with the assistance of her friends/bridesmaids. This just goes to show that not only is one juggling school but also their personal life. That's why it's always important to maintain good time management and a healthy work/life balance.

5

Second Semester

After getting through that first semester, I knew what I struggled with and what I should be more focused on during the upcoming spring semester. I had to remember that not only did I want to do better for myself, but I needed to maintain certain grades in order to keep my scholarship and to still be qualified to continue on with this nursing program. The spring semester consisted of Med-Surg Part II with the clinical, Research Methods, Pediatrics with the clinical the first half of the semester and Maternity with the clinical the second half of the semester. I was really excited to begin this semester because my main population interests were pregnant women and children/babies. However, once the syllabus was available, I knew that my experience would be limited in this area. This was probably the most difficult semester for me because of that. This program was an accelerated program, and having to learn two different areas of nursing within 3.5 months was definitely going to be a challenge.

The Pediatrics lecture portion wasn't as informative as I had hoped. The professor provided way too many slides per PowerPoint (literally over 100) and she read straight from the slides with no extra information to better grasp what was important. So I knew that this semester, any quizzes, tests, or information I didn't understand, I needed to go see my professor after class or during office hours to ask questions. I'm more of a timid individual, especially in class. I'm not the kind of student that raises their hand for every question or sits near or at the front of the class. Plus, our class size was large at times due to the second and first-degree students being in classes together. Most classes were only 45 minutes long, so it was imperative to pay attention. I also went to the library more often, hoping that the difference in the atmosphere compared to being in my apartment, with less distractions, would be more beneficial for me. Lastly, I would attend study groups with other students in my class that may have understood the material better than me, that were better test takers.

These new tactics did help in some ways, at least to keep me above water. This was especially important when it came to the second half of the semester, when it was time to begin the Maternity lecture and clinical. Both Maternity clinical and Pediatric clinical time were very limited; we spent two weekends in clinicals for each of these courses. Unfortunately, when it came to having the opportunity to see an actual birth, I was the only student that never got the chance. Our instructor did random drawings, and being that our clinical time was limited, I never had the honor. Fast forward four months, I was luckily able to see my niece's birth, thanks to my sister's last-minute decision to let me stay in the room while she gave birth. I can honestly say that was such a beautiful moment and I am so glad that I was able to see it.

Although I was doing better with my care plans in my Med-Surg clinical than the first semester, I was struggling to keep my grade at a minimum of a C in my Maternity lecture. Coincidentally, my Maternity instructor was quite informative and succinct with her lectures, which were only 45 minutes. But for some reason, when it was exam time, I just could not deliver. Once we reviewed the answers when we got our tests back, I felt like such an idiot for the questions I would get wrong because I knew what the answer was. At that point, I just needed to make sure my final grade was at least a C. If it wasn't, I wouldn't be able to continue with the program, and I'd have to wait until the following year to repeat that course. That was definitely not a part of my plan, so I knew I had to do the best that I possibly could.

In the meantime, I was chosen by one of my instructors to apply to a student nurse technician position at the Veteran's Affairs Hospital in Baltimore, MD. This position would definitely be perfect for me so that I could start getting that much-needed experience in a hospital. This would allow me to start using what I was learning in the classroom to the actual setting of a nurse. Plus, my sister lived in Baltimore, so that meant I'd have a place to stay close by. After the first semester of core nursing courses, students are eligible to apply for their certified nursing assistant (CNA) license. Thankfully, after turning in the required paperwork and interviewing with the recruiter, I was hired.

The semester was coming to an end, and of course I was anxiety-stricken not knowing if I'd pass. I'd even calculated what I needed to get on the last exam in order to at least pass with a C. I wasn't the only one unsure of passing; there were other classmates that expressed their concerns as well. After getting texts from other classmates saying the exam grades were posted and they'd passed, that only made me even more nervous. By the grace of God, I got just enough answers correct to get a passing grade for the class. I was so relieved, and that summer break was much needed. I couldn't leave school fast enough. Some of the other students who'd worried about passing had barely made it also, except for one of them. I felt so bad for her because if that were me, I'd be a mess and wouldn't know what to do. Of course, you want to see everyone pass with all the studying required and the amount of work we have to do. Fortunately, after speaking with her about it, she was disappointed at first but knowing that she wasn't as passionate to be a nurse as she should be, she came to terms with what had happened. She knew that there was a different life path for her at that moment.

6

Summer Break

S o the summer began, and within a couple weeks I was beginning my new position as a student nurse technician. I had to do the normal hospital orientation during the first couple weeks of starting, then I was able to report to my manager and be assigned my preceptor. My manager was such a sweet, patient older lady, and I was so thankful for the limited time I was able to spend with her. I followed my preceptor's schedule, and on the days she was off, I'd follow another nurse. I was given the choice to either work an eight-hour shift five days a week or work twelve hour shifts three days a week. Being that I wasn't used to working more than eight hours at any job that I've ever had, even when I told myself I would work twelve hours, once that eighth hour hit, I was ready to go home. Also, the shift begins to slow down around that time, making those last four hours seem like forever.

I remember one work shift in particular, where my manager let me float to another unit to get the most of my experience. She sent me to the pre-operative area one day, which was on the same floor as my regular scheduled floor. Overall, the experience was great since I was able to practice starting IVs, but I didn't feel like the nurses were that welcoming. This made me not want to float over there again. However, my manager was retiring, so another manager was in charge of my regular unit until they found a replacement for her. Of course, the covering manager assigned me to go over to that same unit one day. At first, I didn't say anything because I tried to stay positive and try it out again. After a couple hours, I was experiencing the same issues as I had the first time. It just seemed like because the nurses knew that I was still in school and not as experienced as them, they would rather do everything themselves, which made it pointless for me to even be shadowing them for the day. If I couldn't start an IV on the first try, they would just push me to the side and rush to do it themselves. They wouldn't even allow me to try, even if the patient didn't mind that I was still learning. I did speak up and suggest that they let me do more. That was the sole purpose of me being over there, to perfect my skills.

So when this began happening again, I went back to my unit and let the charge nurse know what was going on and that I preferred to be on my original unit than be in the pre-op area. I guess word had gotten back to the covering manager before I was able to speak with her, so she paged me to her office. I had only met her once or twice, and I could tell she was close with one of the nurses that complained about me, so I knew she would be biased. Also, since they were of the same culture/ethnicity, it definitely made me feel uneasy about how they were treating me. I expressed to her what had happened and how it made me feel and that I preferred not to go back over there. As I predicted, she demanded that I go back and didn't take into consideration what I had said. Thankfully, the charge nurse from my regular unit advocated for me and suggested I come back to my regular unit, and I was able to do just that. I appreciated her very much for supporting me. I knew from that day that nurses truly do eat their young, as they say, and this would not be the last time.

7

The Lovely Tales of Home Health

As the summer continued, one of my closest friends told me about a job opening at the company she worked for. She worked for a home health agency and they were looking for CNAs. The job basically included doing whatever daily activities that that particular client needed, whether that be helping with their daily care, household chores, taking them out, etc. I could always use the extra money, and this would only be an as-needed (PRN) job since the hours were variable and depended on the need.

I began this job toward the end of the summer, in August 2012. At orientation, they said that there was a need for a CNA for two hours and that they would be willing to pay $2 extra an hour due to the living conditions of this particular client. Although I was quite nervous, not knowing what to expect, I agreed, and they gave me the assignment. They gave us some supplies that was suggested to keep in your car, such as a box of gloves, and of course the papers we needed in order to document (yes, everything had to be handwritten).

The moment I pulled into the client's development, I could see it was a decent neighborhood, nothing to be on high alert about, being as it was in the morning. I parked in the driveway and got out of the car, and the moment I got to the front door, I could already smell the scent of cigarettes. I have never smoked a cigarette in my life, and I definitely don't like being around the smell of smoke or anyone smoking. So of course I was hesitant, but I had already agreed to do the assignment, and it was only two hours. I knocked on the door and someone hollered from inside telling me that the door was open. The moment I walked inside the house, I saw exactly what my supervisor was talking about. Unfortunately, his house was very disheveled, there was dog feces on the floor and a horrid smell throughout the house, and the floor was barely visible. Being the person that I am, having grown up in a household where everything needed to be clean and tidy at all times, this was quite disturbing to me. I literally was counting the minutes until it was time for me to go while feeling sympathy for this client.

He was bedridden, so he was basically a total care patient. He had a bucket to the side of his bed where he dumped his urine. When I went to dump it in the bathroom toilet, he told me the plumbing system was down so I had to dump it down the sink (yeah, tell me about it). When I went into the kitchen to get him something to eat, there were dirty dishes everywhere, the counters were covered, and the refrigerator had a lot of expired food. All I could do was choose from what food looked and smelled the freshest. The sad part about the whole situation is that his son apparently lived with him and was supposed to be his sole provider, but the home health company felt that the son was taking advantage of his father and living off of his disability benefits.

As much as I felt sorry for that client, I couldn't wait to get out of there. Before I got back in my car, I took my scrub top off, and before I stepped back in my sister's house, I took my shoes off. I couldn't get in that shower fast enough. All I could do is hope that the other clients' homes I visited weren't as unkempt as this one. That's one thing someone taking this job may not consider, as well as the safety factor of going into some random stranger's home. And of course, the wear and tear on your car since you have to have your own transportation. I guess the upside of that is that the company pays you for mileage driven.

After that first client, I went to several other clients' homes before the summer ended. One client's usual caregiver was on vacation, so my supervisor had assigned me to her one day. She barely greeted me when she opened the door for me and didn't seem too fond of me. She was an elderly lady and very particular in her ways. I don't know if maybe she just didn't like that her regular caregiver was out and there were different CNAs coming during this time, or she simply didn't like me for some unknown reason. When it was time to fix her dinner, I asked her what she wanted and prepared her meal the way I would at home as she watched me like a hawk. I usually season my meat on a plate, and she had a comment to say about that but then walked out of the kitchen. As the food was finishing, I asked her what she would like to drink and she told me iced tea with a little bit of sugar. As I was stirring the tea in the cup, one ice cube fell out. Usually when I cook, I taste the food to make sure it's done and seasoned correctly. But I couldn't do that since it was being prepared for her, so all I could do was hope that it was to her liking.

I brought her food and drink to the table, and she took a sip of her iced tea.

I asked her, "How does the tea taste?"

She said, "I guess it's okay. It could've had more ice." Mind you, she was watching when that *one* ice cube fell out.

I responded sarcastically, "Oh, because you wanted that one ice cube that fell out?"

She just ignored me. She proceeded to eat her food but only half of it, and I asked her if the food was to her liking. She told me it wasn't warm enough, that the sweet potatoes tasted like they weren't done all the way. So I said, "Well, how come you didn't tell me when you first tried them? I can warm it up for you if you'd like." She agreed, so I warmed them up. I brought the plate back to her, but she didn't even eat any more. She told me she was finished.

I knew that this woman was going to be a piece of work. Although I was only scheduled to be there for four hours, it felt like an eternity, and I still had two more hours to go. That time couldn't go by fast enough. After dinner, we went into her den and she watched "Little House on the Prairie." We barely spoke during those last couple hours, and I was just so thankful when 8 pm came. When I left, I prayed they'd never asked me to go over there again. It was just so awkward and unwelcoming being there.

A few weeks went by, and I got a call from the home health agency while I was at my SNT job at the VA. They asked if I could go to that lady's house again for a few hours. I told them what had happened the first time I went over there, and they totally understood, but it was last minute, and they couldn't get anyone else. So as hesitant as I was, I agreed to go but told them I might be running a little late since I would be coming straight from my day job.

I was on my way over to her house and I was running behind my start time by 15 minutes, so I called my job to let them know. They said they would call the client to let her know as well. I got to her front door, which had an oval window on the top portion, big enough to see into the home and enough for her to see who was at her front door. I rang the doorbell twice and waited for a few minutes with no answer. I began to become concerned when

I attempted again, so I called my job to let them know. They said they'd try reaching her and would call me back. They called me right back and said that she was home, probably on the other line. So I knocked on the door a few more times. A couple of minutes went by and she walked right in the view of the window, looked me dead in my face, and continued to walk past into the living room. I was totally baffled that this woman literally looked directly at me and chose to ignore me and proceeded to go into another room. So I rang the doorbell until she came to the door.

She opened the door and said, "You're late." I had other thoughts of what I really wanted to say to her but knew I couldn't do that, so I bit my tongue and simply stated, "I apologize for my tardiness, but I let the office know and they said they'd notify you. Plus, I was standing out here ringing the doorbell for the past 10 minutes. You didn't see me when you looked directly at me through the window as you proceeded to walk by?" Of course, she had no answer to that. At that moment, I knew I should've declined this assignment.

It was yet again time for her to eat, and she still seemed to have the same unflattering attitude. As we were at the table, she just gave off a negative vibe like she had a problem with me. This being my job, I wanted to make sure it wasn't anything that I was doing wrong. So I simply asked her, "Do you have an issue with me? I just feel like you don't like me being here."

She said, "Well, you said you didn't like me."

I frowned and said, "Ma'am, I never said those words so please don't repeat something I never said."

Somehow, we came to an understanding, and I just think that she was uncomfortable with having new people coming to her house to care for her. Also, her son was the one who hired someone to come take care of his mother through the week as she clearly needed some assistance. Of course, there could be another reason why she didn't particularly welcome me with open arms. However, from what the office said, all the other CNAs that went over there said the same thing about her. That must've been the reason they couldn't find anyone to go over there for that shift. I was just glad for 8 pm to finally come again, and that was definitely going to be the last time I went over there. There was also a lesson learned in that situation: ALWAYS document what is pertinent, and be careful because there are people that will make up things that are totally untrue just to get you in trouble. From my knowledge, she never went back and told this untruth to my supervisor, but had she, I might have lost my job because of it.

8

Making Connections

As summer 2012 came to a close, I had hoped that I could continue working for both the VA and the home health agency. Thankfully there was an outpatient VA clinic 30 minutes from my school and another office of the home health agency located within the same city as my school. After speaking with the VA nurse recruiter, they were able to get me an interview with the nurse manager at the VA clinic, and she was very impressed with me, so she hired me. The home health agency also gave me the contact information to the nurse in charge at the other office. After meeting with her, they were able to find me a regular client that I saw every Sunday morning for a few hours. Both companies understood that I was still finishing up nursing school and were very lenient when it came to my work schedule. I was able to work at the VA clinic twice a week. I was so grateful to both of them because it allowed me to continue to gain more firsthand experience, hone my skills, and still keep my "foot in the door" in case either one of them wanted to hire me as a registered nurse when that time came.

This final semester of my nursing program was definitely hectic trying to manage two jobs and going to school full-time, not just school, but *NURSING* school. While working at the clinic, I was now able to see a different perspective of working as a nurse.

It was slightly different from the hospital setting because it was obviously smaller, thus allowing a better nurse to patient relationship since those are the same patients that they treat on a regular basis. My shift was from 4-6:30 pm, so by the time I got there, things were starting to slow down. However, no matter what environment you work in, the most critical patient is always first priority. That was witnessed on one of my shifts as we were tending to patients based on their appointment times. One patient in the waiting room started having severe chest pains. Although it wasn't his time yet to be seen, due to his condition, he became the priority patient. He was brought back to the triage area where blood was drawn, an IV line was started, and an EKG was done. Due to his condition and medical history, he was transferred to the nearest hospital by ambulance to better assess and treat him.

Gaining that experience at the VA and getting guidance from all of the nurses was definitely beneficial to my future, as was having to take care of my regular scheduled client through the home health agency. I was assigned to a client that had amyotrophic lateral sclerosis (ALS), also known as Lou Gehrig's disease. He was an older adult who had an angel of a wife. She took such great care of him, and assisted me as well when I came to their home every Sunday. It was the same routine when I came. He slept with a CPAP machine since as this disease progresses, it affects one's ability to breathe effectively. Because I was only a CNA at the time, there were certain things that weren't in my scope of practice to do, so his wife would do it. She would take off the full face mask with hose connection to the CPAP machine and replace it with one that simply went directly to his nose. He would use the urinal and then I'd wash the front of his body by myself. Since the disease progressed, he was only able to slightly move his arms and head, so he wasn't much help when it came to turning him. His wife would then come back in and assist me with turning so I was able to wash his back. After finishing his bath and dressing him, his wife would assist me in transferring him to his automatic wheelchair, using their lift machine. I had never used a lift machine prior to my first day using it with him, only practicing in my nursing skills class.

Once he was transferred and situated in the chair comfortably, he could manage operating the wheelchair himself. His wife would already have his breakfast made by then, and I'd check his blood sugar prior to feeding him. Caring for this client and truly getting to know him and his wife will always resonate with me. They were such humble, respectful, welcoming individuals and appreciated my help. I still think of them sometimes, wondering how they're doing, if he's still alive, if she's alive. That's the conflicting thing with being a healthcare provider. You are taught to achieve good rapport with your patients, but don't allow yourself to get too close to your patients due to the confidentiality component and overstepping that boundary of nurse-patient relationship. That's when you have to have good judgment and make the right decision.

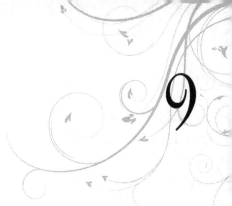

9

Final Semester

This final semester consisted of Psychiatric Nursing lecture and clinical, Community Health lecture and clinical, and Nursing Leadership/Management lecture and clinical. We did our Psychiatric Nursing clinicals at the local hospital where we had been doing our clinicals for the other courses taken during the previous semesters. The hospital had a small 13-bed inpatient psychiatric locked-down unit. We each were assigned a patient to do our assignment on. So the time we spent on the unit, with our instructor present of course, we had to get as much information as possible. The patient I had was a young mother who was suffering from depression. She had been pregnant with twin boys, who were over a year old at this point. Unfortunately, while she was pregnant, she had suffered from a condition called twin to twin transfusion syndrome (TTTS). This meant that one twin was essentially taking up all the blood from the other twin, thus depriving that other twin of essential nutrients to survive in utero. Sadly, that twin died, and the other survived. Due to the loss of one twin, she became depressed because she felt guilty and due to some of her actions, it seemed as though she was detached from the surviving twin.

This was a very interesting case for me because I had already been specifically interested in the maternity aspect of nursing. So this experience gave me the opportunity to experience both maternity and psychiatric nursing. Of course, I was able to witness some of the other patients' behaviors as well. One thing I learned while doing that clinical was that although some may seem to be very "normal" and "sane," you never know what to expect, so your guard should always be up to an extent. Especially since there are some patients with narcissistic behavior that will do exactly what they need to do to build your trust to get what they want out of you.

Of the patients that my class encountered, one was mute possibly from a traumatizing experience, and another was hallucinating. His treatment consisted of trying to figure out if the cause of his hallucinations was truly a psychiatric disorder or if it was more of a medical issue, possibly dementia or Alzheimer's. Our class was also able to sit in on their group meetings to get a better understanding of how the patients interacted with other people, particularly people whom they didn't know while expressing their very personal feelings.

We also witnessed how the nurses passed out their meds, which was of course behind a split locked door at the nurses' station. This was to maintain safety for the staff. And of course, we witnessed an irate patient who at first was quite calm, then began to pace back and forth, and ultimately began acting out. His behavior led the nurses to have to lock down the unit and send the other patients to their rooms in order to maintain safety and calm the situation while they dealt with the patient. We all were behind the nurses' station for our safety.

Overall, my psych rotation was quite interesting. However, I knew that this was definitely NOT the area of nursing that I was interested in or wanted to work in. Little did I know this would not be my last experience with psych.

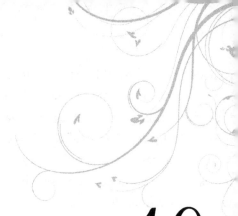

10

Working With the Community

C ommunity health was quite challenging due to the instructor that we had. There were two instructors, who each taught the lecture class together and clinicals separately. They also had very different teaching styles. My clinical instructor gave us more work and definitely wasn't lenient when it came to the quality of our work and experiences for this class.

Even though I loathed that class/clinical, I was very appreciative of the experiences that we had. The first day of clinical consisted of us taking a van ride to different counties in Salisbury. The main purpose was to understand the differences from one neighborhood to the next. By simply looking at the structure of the buildings, lawns, businesses, schools, etc., you just knew whether that neighborhood was low-income vs. high-income. It's sad to say, and it almost seems prejudiced, but this outing actually taught me a lot unbeknownst to my older self. For example, if you see a check cashing store on every block, a Mickey D's, abandoned buildings, and unkempt landscaping, you know that it's a lower income area. When you see an organic food market, nice size family homes, and healthier restaurants, you know that you're in an area that is of higher income. You can also feel whether or not one area is safer than the other. However, no area is exempt from crime.

Besides getting an up close and personal look at the community we were surrounded by, we also took a visit to the detention center. We witnessed how the inmates were housed, what they ate, and the protocol for them to seek medical treatment in the jail. We also walked through both the male and female pods, and of course we had to listen to all of the vulgar, sexual language that they yelled out. We just ignored it as we were instructed to do prior to walking through. I had never taken a tour of a jail or detention center, so it was educational to have that experience. This of course was also a place I definitely did not have an interest in working at in the future either.

The one requirement of this clinical that I did enjoy was the fact that I was chosen to do my volunteer/internship hours at the local health department. Only two of us were chosen to do our hours there, and my other classmates did their hours at a different location. I was even more excited when I was the only one chosen to work with the maternity program within the health department. Once again, I was getting that part of nursing that I was so interested in. I also had very patient and welcoming community nurses to work with. I did home visits with some of the nurses, interviews for prospective Medicaid recipients, and paperwork in the office during any downtime.

When I'd accompany a nurse on a home visit, there were things to pay attention to. The home visits were essential in making sure that not only the mother had the proper tools and resources for a healthy environment for herself and her child, but also to make sure that the child was being properly cared for. It was important to make sure the child was reaching their developmental milestones and getting the proper nutrition. There was one young mother in particular who had a 9-month-old baby, who lived with her boyfriend and mother in a trailer home. Even before entering the home, the community nurse stated that it was important to observe the neighborhood and how the outside of the home was kept. Once inside, I automatically noticed the clutter; there were way too many boxes and miscellaneous items on the floor throughout the home. It almost looked like an episode of hoarders. There was also a cat in the home. Observing this makes you question whether the child is in a healthy environment. All the clutter, and the baby being the age that she was, meant she wouldn't be able to be as mobile as she should be at this age. This meant a possible accident could occur if she did start crawling and an adult took their eye off of her for a few seconds. The cat in the home was also a consideration. No matter how trained a pet can be, they are still an animal with survival instincts, and their behavior can change at any moment. These are definitely things to think of.

However, she appeared to be quite healthy and cared for by her mother. She was a happy baby and appeared to be reaching her developmental milestones. The nurse gave the mother some tips on what to do as far as the house situation and suggestions with learning activities with the baby. She gave her some things to improve on by her next home visit. This was a great experience because these community nurses truly love what they do. They're very personable to these mothers who are simply having some hardships and just need a push to stay on the right path.

Besides doing home visits, I also assisted with office visits of mothers needing assistance. This assistance included WIC, health and dental insurance, and other programs/classes for expectant mothers. There was an interview process that was required to gain more information about the mother and her current situation and future plans. There were two expectant mothers, in particular, that I remember because although their needs were similar, their situations were totally different.

The first expectant mother was a 17-year-old high school student who came in with her mother and her boyfriend's mother. The teenager was about seven months pregnant at this point and was just now reaching out for assistance. While listening to the three of them speak and assessing their situation, it seemed as though the teenager and her mother had a strained relationship. She stated she was currently staying with her boyfriend and his family. It appeared that the teenager was closer to her boyfriend's mother than her own mother. She even stated she hadn't known she was pregnant until recently, which seemed odd because she was very much showing and clearly pregnant. So it seemed as if she knew but was too afraid to tell her own mother, or both mothers were just being oblivious because they didn't want to deal with this teenager being pregnant at such a young age. Also, she was trying to get additional assistance, although she was already covered under her father's insurance, who she didn't even live with. The whole situation seemed odd.

Then there was another expectant mother who was about 22 years old and came in by herself. When asking her the required questions, she had an answer for everything. She had a planner, knew the date of her last menstrual period (LMP), her due date, and she was also still in her first trimester. Being in this interview compared to the other interview was interesting to see how mature and prepared the 22-year-old was compared to the 17-year-old. Not that age matters all the time, but it was clearly evident that the 22-year-old was more mentally prepared for this new baby than the 17-year-old was.

In addition to assisting with the Maternal and Child Health Program, I also shadowed with a nurse who did home visits to adult clients. Some of these adults were disabled or just needed the tools/assistance with programs specific to their needs. One adult in particular we had visited twice. The first time was just a regular visit, making sure she was adjusting well after coming home from the hospital. The second visit was another follow-up, and it was also the last day of my internship. We were only expecting to do a simple home visit, but our assessment of the client showed that her leg wound dressings were saturated. They looked like they hadn't been changed recently. She had a wound nurse, but I guess they hadn't been by, and her live-in adult granddaughter wasn't much help. We couldn't leave her like that, especially since she had methicillin-resistant staphylococcus aureus (MRSA) (just lovely), so that meant I had to assist with the dressing change. After leaving, I couldn't wait to go home and take a hot shower.

Participating in that internship gave me the opportunity to gain a lot of experience with all walks of life and a better appreciation of what the Health Department provides for its community. I was very grateful to have had that, and it gave me another aspect of what the nursing field includes. You can truly see that those nurses weren't in it for the money; they truly cared for their community and those in need.

11

The End is Near

The last half of that final semester of nursing school consisted of our Nursing Leadership and Management lecture and practicum. This course basically consisted of applying all that we'd learned to have a better understanding of the social, economic, legislative, and political forces that have an impact on shaping the United States' healthcare system and the rural environment. The lecture was twice a week as well as the clinical.

Some of our assignments for clinical consisted of speaking with certain leaders of the hospital system, such as the charge nurse, nurse manager, etc., if given the chance, to truly understand their role and how it coincided with other staff members. Everyone has an integral part within the healthcare system, and it was important as nursing students to know what they were and how it affected the system as a whole. Besides that, taking care of our assigned patient(s) became a bit routine and better managed at this point, after having been exposed to all of the other clinicals in previous courses. Of course, this meant our lovely care plans weren't as long as what had been expected in our very first semester's clinical.

At the end of the final semester, we had to take the Health Education Systems, Inc. (HESI) Nursing Exam. This exam was basically a way for the university to see how much we'd learned and how well we had been taught during this program. It was also a taste of what to expect when taking the National Council Licensure Examination (NCLEX); the questions and style of the exam are similar. Most nursing programs require their students to pass this exam; if not, they won't graduate. Luckily, SU did not have this requirement because I surely wouldn't have passed. Although I took the test seriously because I wanted to do well, I didn't get a passing score. However, it let me know that I had a lot of studying to do and what subjects I needed to focus on. I was just so ecstatic that I was going to pass this nursing program. It had been a long, challenging, and stressful journey making it to this point, but I was just so very proud of myself for getting this far. All of my hard work had paid off, and I was one step closer to officially having those letters behind my name (RN). It was time to graduate!

I received the information about the pinning ceremony as well as the day of graduation. Because I had already gone through the graduation process of walking across the stage when I completed my first degree at VCU, I honestly didn't want to do that again. However, the pinning ceremony was most important to me because that was specifically the nursing program's graduation. This was more intimate and special to me, so I decided to attend. I was so thankful for my family for coming to support and celebrate my accomplishments.

We had assigned seating, and as our names were called, we were to walk across the stage, shake our professor's hand, and get our pin. As my name was called, I walked up on that stage and walked across with such pride and courage, knowing that I had been waiting for this joyous day. I smiled as my family took a picture that I will always treasure.

There were light refreshments after the ceremony. We all mingled and met each other's families, and all of the second-degree nursing students took a group picture. Although we were missing a few people from the beginning, we'd still made it!

12

ATL, is that you?

*A*lthough I had completed and graduated from nursing school, the studying wasn't over. The next step was studying for the NCLEX and choosing a date to take the exam. I had already made up my mind that I was going to move to Atlanta, Georgia after graduation. I had never even been there before, but I've always been an adventurous individual, and I wanted a change of scenery. I was young, single, and educated, so what better time than the present to just go for it? Plus, I knew some old friends and people from VCU that had moved there, and of course a guy I was dating lived there. This was definitely not the reason why I wanted to move there, but it was a plus.

About two months prior to graduation, I had made a list of hospitals who had new graduate programs that I was interested in applying to. I had reached out to recruiters to see if they would at least meet with me during my week visit to Atlanta, or a possible interview while there. Luckily, three of them responded and were willing to meet with me. Unfortunately, one of them backed out at the last minute. He told me that he could answer any questions I had through email. But my whole point of meeting in person was so that he could put a name to a face, and I'd actually be remembered when he was looking through all of those applications. However, I still planned to go to that hospital while visiting and speak to a recruiter.

Since I was already working for the VA Hospital, I had hoped that it would be simpler for me to transfer to the Atlanta VA Hospital. One of the recruiters who had been willing to meet with me was from that hospital. Besides meeting with the recruiters, I had plans to meet up with some of the people I knew that lived there, go apartment hunting, and of course enjoy the area to see if this really was the right decision for me.

The week following graduation, I rented a car and made the 10-hour drive by myself to Atlanta. As soon as I hit I-85, it was bumper-to-bumper traffic. This reminded me of DC traffic. This was my first look at what to expect while living in Atlanta.

Although my cousin's friend and husband invited me to stay with them during my trip, I decided to stay with the guy I was dating at the time. I had a busy week ahead of me and was definitely going to make the most of it.

While there, I was able to meet up with old friends, see the nightlife, eat the food, and look at a few apartments. I also was given the opportunity to interview with the VA hospital the day after my scheduled meeting with the recruiter. It was a bit nerve-wracking because I wasn't used to being interviewed by more than one person. I'm already a nervous wreck when I interview with one person, so two people is definitely intimidating. I thought I did well and one of the requirements was to have passed the NCLEX by January 20, 2013.

This gave me about 5 weeks, and it left no room for errors. I also had to consider whether it was a better decision to go for my MD nursing license or my GA license. Luckily the VA takes any state license, and because GA wasn't a compact state and MD was, I thought it'd be smarter to get my MD license. That would give me more options, and I could always apply for a GA license later, if I got a job elsewhere in Atlanta.

In addition to that interview, I also did a shadow day at another hospital in the Medical Intensive Care Unit (MICU). That experience really showed me all of the intricate details and importance of assessments that a nurse must pay attention to. Although that wasn't the type of unit I wanted to work on, I appreciated the opportunity to see it firsthand from a nurse that was recently out of nursing school herself.

Even though I hadn't set up any meetings with any other recruiters from the other hospitals that I was interested in, I at least drove by to see what they looked like or spoke to someone in human resource (HR) about applying.

My week-long trip to Atlanta convinced me that this was the place for me, and I was even more determined to move there. Once I put my mind to something, I don't give up until I get it or it's just out of my reach. I didn't know if I was financially capable to make the move that soon, but I was going to scrape together all the money I had to get there.

NCLEX: Pass or Fail

*I*t was now time to get to studying. Through our Student Nursing Association (SNA), we worked with the NCLEX practice company called Hurst. They set up a week for our class to study with one of their representatives. There was a raffle at one of our SNA meetings, and surprisingly my name was chosen, so I didn't have to pay for the class as long as I got at least 25 students in my class to pay for and attend the study sessions. Although this seemed simple enough, the second-degree nursing class only had 29 students graduating. So that meant literally getting just about everyone to sign up. Mind you, there are other NCLEX prep classes available. Thankfully, I got 25 people to sign up and attend. One less financial strain to worry about. Those classes aren't cheap.

The Hurst practice session was for three days, in which the instructor basically crammed in those three semesters of nursing school. Thankfully, the study book that was provided, along with the eight-hour classes each day, was very descriptive and easy to follow along. I felt like I learned better during this study course than the three semesters of nursing school. Or maybe this study course only enhanced my learning, allowing me to pull out all of those things that I'd already learned and help me understand better. I thought for sure that this would help me pass the NCLEX on the first try.

Once the Hurst study sessions were over, I studied each and every day, since I only had a limited amount of time before my test date came. I used what I learned from HURST and the study book provided, another classmate gave me access to another NCLEX online study option, and of course I took as many practice questions as I could. I still felt a little worried the night before my exam because I had always barely passed my nursing exams or got just below what I needed to pass. The way the nursing exam questions are worded and the choices given can be very confusing and will definitely trick you into choosing the wrong answer. Plus, the only available testing center on the date I chose was in Lancaster, PA, an hour and a half from me. Also, my test time wasn't until the afternoon, which allowed me more time to freak out during the hours leading up to my exam.

I got to the testing center, said a quick prayer to ease my anxiety, and tried to walk in there with confidence. As the instructions were given prior to the start of the exam, the proctor mentioned that each person was not taking the same test. Some people were in there for their real estate license, LPN license, etc. I had to be mindful of that and not let it bother me if they were done before me. Also, the test can cut off at any given moment depending on how well or how badly you are testing. I just tried my best to stay focused on myself and be confident within my answers.

The test began, and at first, I felt like I was doing fine, but then I started getting a lot of those "select all that apply" questions, which made me second-guess myself. I just felt so overwhelmed and unsure of myself. I kept saying to myself that I needed to relax and focus. After so many questions, a screen will pop up asking if you want to take a break and then start where you left off. Instead of choosing to take a break, because I thought it would distract me, I chose to continue. From what I can recall, I think my test cut off at question number 180. At that moment I knew I had failed. Even though no specific cut-off number necessarily means you passed or failed, I just knew I did. I hadn't heard of anyone's test cutting off at such an odd number. The lowest amount of questions you can get is 75 and the highest is 265.

I left that day crying my eyes out on the way home. Not only did I feel confident that I had failed, but that meant that I wouldn't qualify for the nursing position at the Atlanta VA hospital that I had interviewed for the month prior. My dreams of moving to Atlanta were shattered.

I remember calling my friend Shardae, telling her the news. She tried to reassure me that I probably did fine and was just overreacting. She also told me that even if I didn't pass, I could always take it again. I knew she was just trying to be a supportive friend, but I wasn't trying to hear any positivity at that moment. I called my mom and told her also. Once I got back to my sister's (where I was residing at the moment), I tried to see if I'd passed or failed. There's a trick that I learned from others where if you try to sign up again for the NCLEX, the webpage won't let you proceed to the payment screen if you've passed. If you failed, then it will. When I tried it, it let me proceed to the payment screen. That was confirmation to me that I'd failed. It was a Friday afternoon, and there was no real way to guarantee until that Monday whether I'd passed or failed. On top of that, I received an email from the VA stating that they'd chosen another applicant for the position I had interviewed for. That made me wonder if somehow they could already tell that I had failed or if they had simply chosen to go with another applicant. It didn't matter what the reason was; I cried the rest of the evening and began studying again right away.

My sister and brother-in-law tried to cheer me up and told me to stop studying and just take a break and get myself together. I didn't want to hear anything they were saying because all I wanted was that nursing license. I'd fought and studied so hard to get to this point and I was not giving up that easy. This is all I'd ever wanted, and I wasn't going to let one failure decide my future.

I did end up taking a break that night, but when Monday morning came, I was right back on it. I paid the $10 to get the confirmation of whether I'd passed or failed, and of course, I failed, as I'd figured. Unfortunately, you can't retake the test until 45 days later, and of course, you have to pay again. So I signed up for the next available date. I also made sure that the testing center was nearby and in the morning. I knew this time that I needed to mainly focus on the practice questions. I think I was so focused on the content itself and not taking enough practice questions. From that day forward until the night before my second attempt, I made sure to do practice questions all day every day, with no distractions.

The day came when it was time to take my exam again, March 3, 2013. This time I felt more confident in myself and didn't second-guess my answers. Every time the screen popped up asking if I wanted to take a break, I made sure to take that break. This allowed me to regroup and reassure myself that I *was* passing this time, no matter what. As the questions began to go into the 200s, I worried a bit because I obviously knew that the computer felt that I didn't know enough for the test to cut off. At the same time, I was getting enough correct that it wasn't ready to cut off on me. At 265 questions and 6 hours of being in that testing center, the test cut off. I was relieved for it to finally be over but still anxious to know whether I'd passed this time.

As soon as I got home, I did the trick again, and initially it did put me to the payment screen, so I was filled with grief again. But then, when I tried to do it one more time, it wouldn't let me go through. I also looked myself up in the "Lookup A License" section of the Maryland Board of Nurses website and there was my name! I was elated. The hard part was finally over! I was so proud of myself and eager to apply for more nursing positions and finally be in the career I had always hoped for. I couldn't wait to share the news with my family and friends; they were so happy for me.

Just because I had to take the test twice, it didn't make me feel any less knowledgeable than my peers. I knew that I wasn't the best test taker for these nursing exams, but that didn't determine what kind of nurse I was going to be. I had another classmate that failed the first time as well, but I told her what I had gone through and encouraged her to take it again. She ended up passing on the second time as well.

I say this to encourage you to not give up if and when that time comes. I've heard of others having to take the test five or six times, but they never gave up. That type of drive and determination lets you know how much you want it. Don't let one failure discourage you or determine your future. There are so many people in this world who've had setbacks, but remember, "the comeback is always greater than the setback." If being a nurse is your true passion, your time *will* come.

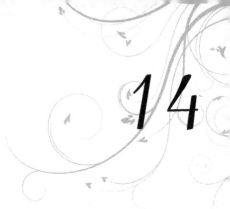

14

Job Search

Upon receiving my nursing license, it was now time for me to start applying for nursing positions again. Since my Atlanta move had fallen through, my plans were now to stay in Maryland. Since I had already been staying with my sister in Baltimore and working as a CNA for a home health agency, I decided to apply to hospitals in and around Baltimore. My first thought was to apply at the VA hospital since I had already been working there as a student nurse technician while in nursing school. I still had the nursing recruiter's information, so I attempted to contact her several times to no avail. Thankfully, I was still called in for an interview for the position I had applied for.

There were four people interviewing me (very nerve-racking) who asked questions based on my education, specifically about the cardiac system since it was a cardiac floor. I'm always nervous when it comes to interviewing, but I did my best to answer their questions, express my willingness to learn as a new nurse, and ask them questions as well. They made me feel so confident that they were going to hire me; they gave me a tour of the unit as well. Unfortunately, I got my hopes up. After trying to follow up with them a few times, I hadn't heard anything back and assumed that they'd hired someone else for the position.

So there I was on the search again. While applying for other positions, I also attended a nursing job fair that one of my nursing classmates was attending as well. I made sure to bring enough copies of my resume and cover letter to give to all of the places I was interested in. Make sure you always carry extra copies just in case; you always want to be prepared for anything. Going to these job fairs can be intimidating because you are one of hundreds of applicants, and it's even more intimidating to be a new nurse. Some companies aren't as eager to hire someone new because that takes time and money; they'd rather have someone that already knows what they're doing. On the other hand, there are some that would love to hire new nurses to mold and train. However, it is imperative to make sure you stand out somehow when going to these job fairs; to make yourself known, make eye contact while speaking to the recruiters so that they'll remember you.

I made sure to do just that, specifically with one recruiter who I was able to have a one-on-one conversation with. I'm usually a shy person when it comes to conversing with others who I do not know, but in situations like these, I have no choice but to speak up and let my voice be heard. Although it was brief, I made sure to make an impression on her, and she let me know what new nurse positions were available and encouraged me to apply. She said to contact her directly by email when I had applied. That very moment led me to my first nursing job. Shortly after applying, I was called in for an interview. The position was for a psychiatric/ behavioral health nurse. Although I wasn't thrilled about working on that unit, I took it as an opportunity. I just needed to get my foot in the door somewhere, and I didn't want to still be without a nursing job months later.

15

The Real Psych 101

I interviewed with the nurse manager of that unit the day of my interview. He stopped the interview at one point because he could tell that I was a bit nervous and gave me a tip after observing something that I was doing. He told me to just relax, be myself, and to make eye contact. I didn't realize that I tend to look away when speaking in an interview; it's just me being nervous. At the end of the interview, I made sure to ask him how he felt about my interview and if he was considering anyone else. He was surprised that I had asked that but was impressed by it. He told me he had another candidate, and that I had done well. Within 24 hours of my interview, I made sure to send a succinct thank-you email to him, making sure to add something we'd spoken about in the interview. He replied, and within the next few days I received notification that I got the position! I was ecstatic but also so very thankful that someone took a chance on me. By the way, he did mention that my thank-you email sealed the deal (hint, hint).

Of course, being a new nurse, that meant only 12-hour night shifts were available. Most new graduate positions only have night shifts or rotating shifts available. You have to have a few years under your belt or be a seasoned nurse in order to choose the shift you prefer. Although I had no choice but to choose a night shift, I'd at least be getting paid a differential on top of my regular pay.

So there was some positive to working night shift. I was assigned a day shift and night shift nurse preceptor. I did three weeks of dayshift so that I could get an idea of what occurs during dayshift as opposed to nights. My dayshift preceptor was a fairly new nurse herself and about the same age as me so she was able to give me advice on some things. It was a little easier to relate to her because she had just been in my position a short year prior. It was definitely a struggle staying awake while working a 12-hour shift since I had never done this before, but I soon got the hang of it.

Working on a psych unit was definitely challenging and mentally exhausting at times. There are patients of all ages, ethnicities, and walks of life. These patients are not only suffering from a mental condition but also have medical conditions that need monitoring. But as long as those medical conditions were stable, they were on our unit to monitor and treat their mental conditions. There were protocols we needed to abide by while treating these patients. This was a locked unit, as most psych units are, to protect the patient so that they don't just decide to walk off the unit. Although there were two sets of double locked doors to get in and out of the unit, it still needed to be monitored because there were times that a patient would attempt to leave the unit by following close behind someone authorized to enter and exit.

Once admitted to the unit, patients were only allowed two outfits during their stay, no belts, nothing sharp, no lighters/weapons/smoking (of course), none of their own bath/beauty products from home, and of course the preliminary paperwork needed to be done. There were those employees that cut corners and allowed certain products at times, which made it difficult when someone like me needed to enforce the rule. The protocols needed to be followed for the safety of the patients and the staff;

any minor break in that rule could possibly lead to harm. There were limited visiting hours for family members, and during this time, anything the family brought in had to be placed in a locker. The hospital security officers were present during this time to make sure nothing was brought onto the unit that wasn't allowed. This was also a time to be vigilant of any suspicious activity since there were more people to account for and monitor. Although these protocols were in place, there were still times when things would get past the staff.

There were various patients admitted for many different reasons. Some truly needed help due to a psychotic break or a distinctive event that caused them to become depressed to the point they were considering suicide. There were also those who didn't necessarily need any mental health treatment. They may have just stated they were suicidal/homicidal because they needed some place to shower, eat, and sleep for a few days. There were also times when the psych doctors weren't exactly forthcoming when it came to their patients. By that, I mean some would convince their regular patients to make false accusations to get admitted so the doctor could get paid, and in turn, that patient would get medicated. There were also times when a patient might have been well enough to be discharged, but instead the doctor would keep them longer to get paid. When the nurses called to get orders for a newly admitted patient in the middle of the night, the doctor sometimes asked us, "Well, what do you think?" or "Just put the same orders in from last time." I would think to myself, "Um, I'm not the one with the medical degree. Although I appreciate you asking my input, these decisions are ultimately on you, not me." Doctors will also throw a nurse under the bus to save themselves, even if they were the one in the wrong. Always get clarification from the doctor and document it verbatim.

Witnessing these situations firsthand really opened my eyes up to the healthcare field. It showed me that it is truly a business and saddened me because this was not what I signed up for. Despite that, I promised I would always keep the vow I'd made when getting that nursing license; that I would do my job because I was passionate about it, not because of a paycheck. I wouldn't allow myself to fall in that "bad apple" category because this was not the type of job where you can slack off, even for a minute. These are people's lives that you are responsible for, and even after you clock out for the day/night, anything that happened on your shift that is a direct result of negligence will still fall back on you.

Caring for these patients meant being alert at all times, never letting your guard down. There were patients that made passes at me/flirted with me, cussed me out, tried convincing me to give them PRN medications that they clearly did not need, and those who tried but failed at being physically violent with me. No matter how relatable a patient may be, you have to always remember that they are the patient and you are the nurse. There still has to be a professional boundary, and you must not forget that.

There were also those patients that I truly felt sorry for because they needed more one-on-one attention. For example, there was a lady who suffered from a traumatic brain injury (TBI) after falling down the stairs because she drank a lot. Her family felt she needed to be admitted because of her recent erratic behavior. However, I just felt that this particular unit wasn't the place for her. Being that she didn't have the same brain function as someone without a TBI, it was difficult with her being on the unit. She required more attention and followed the staff around a lot while crying because her reactions were more childlike. Thankfully she wasn't on the unit too long.

16

Older Nurses Eat Their Young

*B*esides maintaining alertness with the patients, it was also important to do this with the other staff members. The old saying "Older nurses eat their young" is unfortunately very true. During the first few months of working on that unit, I got along with pretty much all the staff. Some I didn't particularly care for, but I didn't allow that to affect the professional relationship I had to maintain to still have an effective work environment. There was one nurse in particular that my preceptor and some other staff warned me about, but of course I never allow others' opinion to cloud my judgment toward people I do not know. However, I make sure to make note of what they say so I am prepared for if and when the same situation arises for me. Let's refer to her as "Nurse G."

I would see her have disagreements and mild arguments with some of the other nurses about small, petty things. One time she got upset with my preceptor because my preceptor was simply showing her the correct way to do an EKG. I guess Nurse G felt as if my preceptor was talking down to her, and she somehow felt embarrassed. So instead of taking the advice and applying it so she would know next time what to do, Nurse G chose to argue with my preceptor. Then there was a time when I received an email from my manager reminding me that it is unprofessional for me to be on my cell phone while at the nurses' station. Although in any job setting, using your personal phone while on the clock is prohibited, most people do it anyway. I saw several staff members doing it and might have even seen my manager at one point, but instead of disputing it, I just took heed and made sure not to do it. At this point, I knew someone must've told on me, because there was no way that my manager had personally seen me on my phone. This made me very cautious around my co-workers, especially since I was still fairly new.

I had just finished my orientation and was now on my own with my own set of patients. I was nervous but confident that I knew enough to do my job and any questions I had I could ask one of the other nurses. I came in one night and had to get a change of shift report from Nurse G. Although I questioned her about much of the report she gave me, I was fresh off of orientation and she was a seasoned nurse, so I felt a bit inferior in my confidence. It's important to always remember to ask questions. Don't let the fact that someone is more experienced than you make you think that your questions are irrelevant. As you become more skilled, and with the proper guidance, you'll know what questions are imperative to ask and which ones you can figure out the answers to yourself. Especially with a nurse like her, you should always double check before the off-going nurse leaves. Once they clock out, you are now responsible. Little did I know that night would be a turning moment in my thought process and the way I viewed other nurses.

As I was looking at each patient's chart, I could see plenty of things Nurse G never did. There were two diabetic patients, one of whom was recently admitted during day shift. I noticed there was no documentation of either patient's glucose level being checked. Although the patient nurse technician (PCT) would normally check a patient's glucose level, it is ultimately the nurse's responsibility to make sure that it is completed. This concerned me because if these two patients had abnormal levels, this would now fall on me since they were now in my care. Thankfully, their glucose levels weren't abnormal to the point of an emergency and requiring notifying a physician. There was also a third patient, who had multiple STAT doctor's orders from 2 pm on day shift while Nurse G was their nurse and clearly signed off on seeing the orders. However, they were never done, so now I had to do them. What made it look bad is that they were now being done 6+ hours later. Thankfully, I had a co-worker working with me that night that I could always turn to for assistance, and she helped me get everything done.

She even told me I should document what wasn't done prior to my shift to cover myself in the future. I was listening to her but at the same time I didn't want to get anyone in trouble. That mentality changed very quickly. At about 1 am during my shift, the phone rang, and guess who it was—Nurse G. Now why in the world would she be calling at 1 am, especially when she was scheduled to come back into work at 7 am? Instead of speaking to her, I passed the phone to another nurse. After getting off the phone with her, the nurse told me that Nurse G was inquiring about whether the orders that she'd decided *not* to do had been completed. While asking that, she decided to tarnish my reputation and make up lies about how I wasn't a good nurse and didn't do my work. This caught me by total surprise. I didn't understand where this was coming from, but all I could think of was what everyone else had warned me about. The only reason Nurse G called was because she had a guilty conscience about not completing what she was supposed to complete and was just trying to cover herself.

I made sure to document everything that happened so that I could have it ready to send to my manager when he came in that morning. Plus, I had a witness that was willing to vouch for me. Before I left to go home, my manager had a meeting with me, Nurse G, and the other nurse who would be my witness. It took every ounce in me to bite my tongue and not scream at the lies Nurse G was telling when she told her side of the story. I just knew from that moment on, never trust anyone because when you least expect it, there will be someone willing to throw you under the bus. While driving home after the meeting, my manager called to reassure me that he trusted me, believed in me, and that he'd made the right decision in hiring me, and to never let someone else beat me down. With that being said, it gave me confidence in knowing that without him exactly saying it that he knew that Nurse G was lying and this wasn't the first incident with her. Unfortunately, she still had her job, but I wasn't going to allow her to diminish what I had worked so hard to accomplish. From that moment on, I learned a very valuable lesson: *ALWAYS* document, not only on your patient but your coworker. You never know when an issue will arise, and you need something to corroborate your story. This very lesson prepared me for future incidents where I had to defend myself and my license.

17

Change is Near

I continued to work on that unit for the next 11 months. While gaining as much experience as I could, I was also looking for another job that would allow me to truly use my nursing skills. I yearned for that kind of experience, and working on a behavioral health unit wasn't going to get me it. On top of that, working on that unit was beginning to be stressful with being short-staffed, no male coworkers to assist with the unruly patients during night shift, and working with coworkers who weren't willing to help each other. However, I didn't realize how difficult it would be to transfer to another unit with only having behavioral health experience. I had applied to several hospitals in the area, and no one would even call me for an interview. I even considered travel nursing because of how much more money you can make. Who wouldn't want to see the world while making good money?

Since I wasn't getting any interviews, I began calling some of the HR departments of the hospitals that I had applied to. I was able to speak with a lady from one hospital's HR department and express my concerns about my application and what could possibly be the reason I kept getting rejected. She simply told me it was because I only had behavioral health experience, and I wasn't considered a "brand new nurse" after working for almost a year, so I was in a gray area. This information discouraged me because I felt like I'd never at least get a call for an interview for me to at least prove to them how badly I wanted a change and how much of an asset I could be. Thankfully, she gave me a chance and scheduled me to come in for an interview for a cardiac unit that was hiring. After the interview and doing a walkthrough of the unit, I felt very confident about getting the job, and HR even called me to tell me that I was chosen for the job. Unfortunately, they'd gotten the applicants mixed up, and it was actually another nurse that got the job. I was even more upset about the fact that they'd gotten my hopes up, but I wasn't going to stop looking. I just looked at it as maybe that position wasn't meant for me.

One of my coworkers, A.M., applied for a transfer within our hospital to a medical-surgical/telemetry floor. She told me that she'd met with the hiring manager, and she said she'd put in a good word for me as well since they had a couple of other open positions available. I was beyond thrilled because whether I wanted to stay at that hospital or not, I would at least get my foot in the door to get the experience I had been wanting. Of course, another nurse that we worked with, who started working on our unit after me, heard of the open position on the med-surg/tele unit as well and applied. That's another reason you can't always trust your coworkers; some of them are always in competition with you and trying to steal your shine.

A.M. had already put in a good word for me to the hiring manager, so I just had to do my part in reaching out to her. Unfortunately, after trying to call her on two or three different occasions and leaving a voicemail, I could never reach her, and she never returned my call. Thankfully she came on the unit one day, and A.M. introduced us so I was able to set up a time to meet with her. Honestly, if she hadn't just happened to come on our unit when she did and if A.M. wasn't there to take the initiative to introduce us, I probably wouldn't have ever gotten the opportunity. As I stated previously, always make your voice heard no matter what. I had figured the nurse manager had gotten my calls/voicemail but just wasn't interested in speaking with me, so it discouraged me. However, I truly believe that everything happens for a reason, and there was a reason she came on that unit that day and A.M. was there for me.

After I spoke with her, she asked when I was able to sit down with her for an interview. We scheduled a day and time to meet. Although this time was literally right after I clocked out after working a 12-hour night shift, I couldn't make any excuses. If you really want something, you can't let anything stand in your way. I was exhausted, but I was *still* going on that interview.

Our interview went well, and she set up a time for me to shadow one of the nurses for four hours so that I could get a feel of the unit and see how well I'd fit in on the unit and with the staff. Once that was complete, I'd know whether or not I got the position. Thankfully all went well with shadowing the nurse and I was hired! I was so elated to have this opportunity and finally start using what I learned in nursing school in the real world.

18

Med-Surg/Tele

My preceptor during my orientation period was the same nurse I had shadowed with. We got along well, we are about the same age, and she was definitely the right choice, similar to the two preceptors I'd had while on the behavioral health unit. This unit was totally different from what I had been used to for the past year. Of course, mental illness also affects people with medical illnesses, so I'd still encounter patients that exhibited the same symptoms as those I cared for on my previous unit. However, the difference was that these patients, whether they had a mental illness or not, were solely admitted to this unit due to other health illnesses. The patients on this unit ranged from withdrawing from drugs/alcohol to those who were total care on ventilators. The patients on ventilators always worried me a bit because they were solely dependent on a machine to breathe for them, so they required more attention to detail. Although the respiratory therapists were there to do their daily rounds on any patient with respiratory related needs, it was still up to the nurse to do their part as well.

Thankfully I had a great preceptor, so those six weeks of orientation truly prepared me as much as possible prior to being on my own. But of course, the one thing you didn't learn during orientation comes up when you're on your own. An example of this happened when I was only about a week off of orientation. The charge nurse from the day shift, who made the night shift assignment, didn't make a great decision when she made my assignment. I had four assigned patients that night, two of which were older patients with dementia who'd both just had their sitters discontinued earlier that day. A sitter is someone who is assigned to watch the patient at their bedside throughout their entire shift due to the unpredictable behavior of the patient. It's an extra safety measure to keep the patient from harming themselves and/or others. There are specific positions for someone who wants to strictly just be a sitter. If one is not readily available, a PCT is assigned to sit with the patient for their shift, or a nurse if staffing is really short.

Unfortunately, I was quite busy earlier in my shift, doing med pass while assessing each patient, and one of the two older patients who had been recently taken off of a sitter had attempted to get out of bed. While doing so, he was attached to a continuous IV and a urinary catheter. He was obviously still confused, and the sitter was prematurely discontinued. He unfortunately had a fall, but thankfully my preceptor was scheduled to work that night, and she was able to assist before I got to the room. When a fall occurs, there is a protocol to follow. First, you need to assess the patient and take vitals, make sure to check for any new scrapes, bruising, or pain. Then you need to notify the on-call doctor. Usually the doctor will order lab work and most importantly, a head CT scan and any other necessary X-rays, depending on how the patient fell. It's important to cover everything to check for anything internally problematic that can't be seen on a simple assessment. The charge nurse of course needs to be notified so that there's an extra precaution in place for this patient now being a high fall risk. Next, you have to do a succinct documentation in the patient's chart of what occured and fill out an incident report. The incident report gives a short synopsis of what occurred, who was notified, what was ordered, and if any initial injury was noticed on assessment. The purpose of the incident report is to build data for the hospital to see how frequently certain incidents occur and what solutions can be implemented to prevent such from occurring in the future. Additionally, anything that happens during the patient's stay that isn't a direct result of the patient's illness and something that could've been prevented falls back on the hospital. Insurance companies will not cover those costs.

Unfortunately, this patient suffered a fractured leg from the fall, and due to the severity, a resolution meeting had to be held. I was worried for the patient, especially because a fracture at his age was serious, and it lengthened his hospital stay. It wasn't mandatory for me to go to the resolution meeting since there were going to be two other nurses representing my unit, but my manager thought that it would be beneficial for me to go. I also thought it was important for me to be there so that I could have a better understanding of what occurs in these incidences and the fact that he was my patient, so I felt responsible. The attendees included members in higher-up management, the two nurses from my unit and myself; there were about 10 of us in the meeting. We basically discussed the statistics of falls worldwide, in our region, and specifically within our hospital. We also discussed the effect it has on the patient and the hospital, and particularly the incident at hand.

I explained what had occurred as I'd witnessed it, and we discussed different scenarios in which this could have been avoided and what should be implemented for the future. One issue in particular is that the patient had a Posey (fall alarm) on, but it wasn't set up to my nurse work phone as it should have been. When the alarm is programmed in the computer to your hospital cell phone correctly, an alert should go off when the patient makes the slightest movement off of the pad. I never received an alert that he was getting out of the bed. Another nurse just happened to walk by the room and heard the alarm from the Posey itself, which notified her that he was out of bed. At this point, it was too late. However, another precaution would be to put a bed alarm on. Most hospital beds have a bed alarm button you can set, which will also alert someone if the patient gets up.

This incident was definitely a learning experience for me. It was unfortunate that it took such a drastic incident, but thankfully the patient eventually healed and was discharged from the hospital. The takeaway from this is to know that nursing isn't perfect, and mistakes happen in every profession. It is imperative to think ahead and always triple check yourself. Some things are inevitable and out of your hands, but the things you can help prevent make sure to do so. The slightest mistake could cause you your license, or in an extreme case, a lawsuit and criminal charges.

19

The Grass Isn't Always Greener

I also had problems with some of the older nurses on this unit as well. I could tell you several incidents that occurred. One nurse in particular had worked with me on night shift and chose to always give me the first admission or one that was particularly difficult. I usually bite my tongue, so to speak, and observe the situation, and if I feel like I'm being targeted I speak up and try to resolve the situation with the person before going to a supervisor or manager. There was a night when once again, I felt like she was picking on me, giving me an admission when she really should've taken it. She felt that because she was the charge nurse that she shouldn't take it. However, everyone else already had about four patients, and she only had two or three. She made a big scene about it so I made sure to let my manager know that morning how I felt about the other nurse. Surprisingly, my manager said she had been waiting for me to come to her about this nurse. She said that my former preceptor and other staff had mentioned how the nurse was treating me but wanted me to come to her about it myself. It was refreshing to know that I wasn't alone in this and it had been witnessed by others. From that point on, I didn't have any more issues with her.

I also had a few mishaps with a seasoned nurse who half-assed her work as well. She was an older lady and had been an LPN for years. She was near retirement, and every time I got report from her, there was always something she didn't do. Once again, being fresh off orientation, I didn't particularly always know what things to check before the off-going nurse clocked out. This night in particular, she was supposed to give one of her patients a blood transfusion that was ordered on her shift, way before I had come in. She had not started it, or even gone to get the blood. I saw the doctor's order in the patient's paper chart and consulted with my preceptor about it. She confirmed that I needed to talk to the off-going nurse about that order because it should've been her responsibility to start the blood, especially since that is not something that should be delayed. Luckily that nurse didn't leave yet for the day, and we'd both inquired about why it had not been given. Due to the fact that I had another nurse with me that the seasoned nurse knew better than me, that seasoned nurse did what she *should've* already done instead of putting that order on to me. Otherwise, she would've made it my problem. This was yet another incident that could be very detrimental to the patient if not carried out as soon as possible, and it could've been my butt on the line, since I already had taken report from her and was about to sign off on checking that chart. That particular nurse actually ended up getting fired—well, she was offered to resign due to a list of incidents, so she would still get whatever retirement benefits were available to her.

By the way, most hospitals have predominantly electronic charting. This particular hospital had an ancient electronic medical records (EMR) system, including a lot of paper charting. So when we checked the patient's chart, we had to sign off after the last order or signature that we had checked the chart, with a date and time.

Up until this point in my nursing career, I had other coworkers who experienced their patients dying or having near death experiences. However, I had never actually had my own experience of a patient dying, nor did I ever want to, but this is a field where it's almost inevitable not to experience this at some point in your career. It was a man in his 60s, who was being transferred from the ICU floor to our floor. I was the one who took the report from the ICU nurse to admit him during this shift, and he was my patient the very next night as well. We already knew that he was on comfort care because his health was to the point where there was nothing left to do to prolong his life. Comfort care is basically making the patient as comfortable as possible in their last days, hours, minutes, and seconds. Usually that includes giving pain meds such as morphine, suctioning their mouth if necessary, and just meeting their daily hygiene needs.

This gentleman had a history of alcohol abuse amongst other illnesses which ultimately led to liver failure. This in turn, caused all his other organs to shut down. Upon assessment, his whole body was swollen due to the increased fluid, he didn't respond to anything I said, and he only opened his eyes occasionally. Although he couldn't verbally respond to me, I still introduced myself as I always do. I let my patients know I will be the nurse for this shift, make sure their call bell is in reach, and always inform them of any care I am about to do or any medication I am going to give them. It is so important to build a good rapport with your patients because you have to remember that they are there alone. We don't know all the emotions or struggles they may be facing, and by showing them true compassion and empathy, it builds a better relationship and trust.

I only took his vitals at the beginning of the shift to get a baseline of where they were. Usually, standard vitals are taken every four or eight hours; of course it depends on the patient. Since he was comfort care, there was no need to keep taking them throughout the shift. I particularly paid attention to his respiration rate because he was breathing very slowly. Normal respiration rate on a healthy individual is 12 to 20 breaths per minute. His was about six; he had what they call agonal respirations. It is a reflex of the brainstem, getting out your last gasps. I had never seen someone breathe that slowly or go through the dying process, so this was very new to me. I felt a bit uneasy in that moment because I did not want to experience that on my shift.

After I left his room, I went to check on my other patients. At one point as I passed by his room, I noticed he had a visitor. I was actually shocked because from viewing his chart and getting report from the nurse who transferred him, he apparently never had any visitors. What shocked me even more is I noticed he was moving his arms around and he was trying to communicate, but he hadn't exhibited any of this while I was in the room with him. He was a complete vegetable for me, but I guess being around a familiar face gave him any last bit of energy his body possessed to respond. I went in to introduce myself, and the woman told me she was his daughter. She had called another family member and had the phone on speaker so her dad could communicate with them.

In that moment, I felt a sense of warmth, because I knew that man was going to die soon, and I knew how important that moment meant to him and his family members. He had a burst of energy, and that energy made so much sense moments later. The daughter left shortly after. I didn't see her leave because I was with my other patients, but I would periodically check in this man's room to make sure he was still alive, basically. I peeked into his room and I noticed he was kind of convulsing and bringing up more sputum than he had been before. I was occasionally suctioning his mouth because his secretions kept building up since he couldn't swallow very well on his own. They were clearer secretions before, but now it was like an orange color and a lot more coming out. I knew that this was it; he was dying right in front of me, and there was nothing I could do because he was a DNR, or Do Not Resuscitate. That means that no matter what, you cannot perform CPR, cardiopulmonary resuscitation. This is based on the patient's wishes, family or healthcare power of attorney for that patient if the patient doesn't have the mental capacity to make such a decision.

It is important to know whether your patient is a full code (they want CPR) or is a DNR. If you perform CPR on a patient that is a DNR, you will be liable because at that point you are going against their wishes, and that will open up a lawsuit, especially if that person indeed comes back to life. You can find this order in the patient's paper chart, electronic chart, and they should have a DNR hospital wristband.

I had asked one of the other nurses to come in the room with me, and I told her that he was a DNR. She stayed there while I called the doctor on call, because the doctor is the one who has to document the time of death. When she came to the room, I had his paper chart in hand so she could confirm everything. There was a question at one point if he was a full code and if we should do CPR because there was a form in his chart that said he was a full code, but everywhere else was saying DNR. We were able to clarify this immediately. That is definitely not something you want to be unsure of in a life or death situation because every second counts.

She checked his breath sounds with her stethoscope, checked his pulse and announced his time of death. The next steps were to prepare his body to be transported to the hospital morgue, notify the family, and of course document. The doctor has their own paperwork to fill out and sign, including the death certificate, and this has to be included with the patient's chart. So two coworkers and I started preparing him to be transported. We had to remove his urinary catheter, clean him up, put a fresh gown on him, and put a toe tag on to identify him. He also had a central line in his chest, but the doctor was responsible for removing that. After all that was complete, we had to put him in a body bag and transfer him onto the mortuary bed. We all then transported him to the hospital morgue.

After all that was completed, I was finally able to document everything and tend to my other patients. That moment makes you appreciate life and humbles you because you never know when your time is coming. Looking back, I now understood why the patient all of a sudden was moving around and trying to talk when his daughter came. It's almost like he was waiting, and he used his last bit of energy in that moment with her. That's special. I always heard of situations where someone was going to die but they held on until a certain person or people came to see them before they took their last breath. It's amazing how life works and how your body responds in different situations. Although this was a sad situation to watch, I am glad I got the opportunity to be a part of it and experience it. Nursing is not just about caring for the sick and keeping a person healthy; it's also about comforting that person in their last moments and even after death. I didn't know that man or his past, but that's none of my business. My job was to do exactly what I did, and I'm satisfied with how I handled it.

After gaining almost a year's experience of working on a med-surg/tele unit (basically a stepped-down ICU, but who's being picky), I felt like it was time for a change. Since the plan was never to live in Baltimore after graduation, I still wanted to experience a different atmosphere. I really wanted to try travel nursing because of the pay—and who wouldn't want to travel the world while getting paid doing it? I was single with no obligations, and I felt this would be the perfect time to try it. I knew from talking to other travel nurses that it was important to really hone your skills, be stern about what you deserved to be paid, and be mindful of the location and hospital an agency would be sending you to. All of these aspects were important because an agency can very well screw you over because they're just trying to put you wherever the need is. (I'll give you an example of this later in the book.)

After a couple months of negotiating with travel agencies, I came to the conclusion that it just wasn't for me. It seemed like most of the available positions were in some remote location in different states that I wasn't looking forward to being in. I'd envisioned Miami, Atlanta, Los Angeles, etc. I didn't want to take the risk of taking an assignment somewhere and absolutely hating it, and having no choice but to stay until my contract ended. The lengths vary, but I'd want to do at least a three-month contract. If the contract wasn't fulfilled, you'd be responsible to pay the money back. So my next option was to just move to another city. I didn't really want to move to another state anymore because at this point, I didn't want to be far away from my family. So I decided I'd rather just move closer to Washington, D.C. It was about 45 minutes from where I was currently living. I'd be experiencing a new city while still being close to family. Plus, my apartment lease was ending soon, so I needed to make a decision whether I'd renew or not.

After applying to several hospitals, I ended up getting a call from a recruiter at a hospital in Silver Spring, MD to set up an interview. I was beyond excited because this was actually the hospital I wanted to work at. Since it was an observation unit, I figured it wouldn't be as laboring as what I'd already been doing (I should've known better, but we'll get into that soon). I went to my interview, and I felt really confident afterward, especially since the assistant manager was also an alumnus of VCU. It's always good to have something you and the interviewer can relate to, something they'll remember you for that makes you stand out, as I've stated previously. They specifically told me that the most patients a nurse receives is five, but it could be lower. Since this was an observation unit, that meant patients get admitted and discharged around the clock. The patients seen on this unit were there for health issues that could quickly be ruled out—if not, they'd be sent to another unit for better monitoring (obviously, that didn't turn out to be true). I was also told that there were four nurses scheduled each day and that there were only 19 beds. There were two extra beds available in case of an overflow, but they weren't in rooms, just a curtain for privacy. That being said, I felt pretty comfortable about this being a possible good change for me. They invited me back to do a share day with one of the nurses on the unit to see how well I'd fit in and so I could get a feel of what to expect on a regular shift.

I knew that as long as the share day went well, I definitely had the job. The day I went in for the share day, there were only three nurses (one had called out of course), and every bed was full (go figure!). That meant two nurses had six patients, and one had seven patients. I should've known then that this was a sign to not walk, but run! However, being a nurse and understanding the dynamics of working in the hospital, I knew that this could happen sometimes. Some days are really hectic, and sometimes you're short staffed. It happens. I tried to rationalize the situation because I wanted to leave Baltimore so badly. Additionally, the nurse I was following that day was about to discharge two of her patients, but that meant she'd be admitting some more also. And of course, when the assistant manager talked to me after my four hours were over, she made sure to tell me that the unit was not always like that. She said that it was just one of those days. She said anything she had to in order to ease my worry and not scare me off.

I should've listened to my gut and kept on my job search. However, I knew that this was not the unit I wanted to stay on forever. I really just needed to get my foot in the door, doing something I already knew how to do, then put in a transfer for Labor and Delivery (L&D). My true passion was always to work on an L&D floor, so that was my plan. Little did I know it wouldn't be that simple.

While at work about a week later, I had a missed call and voicemail from the same recruiter with a job offer. I was so ecstatic and called her back immediately. This job offer came right on time because I had just been debating with my apartment rental office whether or not I was going to re-sign my lease. It had been a day after the deadline for me to re-sign and I chose not to, so this job offer had to come through, and it did just that. I simply thanked God and once again He showed me that He is always on time.

My start date was at the end of April, so I had about three weeks to find an apartment close to my new job. Although my current lease wasn't ending until the end of May, there's no way I was commuting from Baltimore to Silver Spring for work. That would be about an hour's drive, not including traffic. Unfortunately, that meant paying for another full month of rent and utilities for an apartment I wasn't going to be living in, on top of paying for a new apartment.

Thankfully, I was able to find one on short notice. My rent was an extra $300 a month compared to what I was previously paying in Baltimore, but that was to be expected being in Montgomery County. At least my pay was increasing by almost $5 an hour (the first increase in my pay in two years of being a nurse), so it all evened itself out. However, the apartment itself, the neighborhood, and the people working in the rental office were a complete and utter disaster, but that's another story in itself.

20

Observing the Chaos

The first week of my new job consisted of orientation, signing paperwork, getting accustomed to the hospital, and listening to representatives' speeches from each department—the usual when starting a new job. The very first day consisted of signing paperwork, which included a "New Graduate Nurse" contract. This basically is what all hospitals require a new nurse to sign nowadays. It's basically a piece of paper forcing you to sign your life over, stating that you have to be on that specific unit or equivalent within the hospital for a specific amount of time or you'll have to pay the hospital back a specified amount of money. This is just the hospital's way of covering themselves if a nurse decides to leave prematurely; the hospital doesn't want to feel like they wasted their time and resources on this one nurse, so they charge the nurse for it. However, no one knows how well they're going to do in a position or if that is even the right choice for them. So you almost feel trapped by signing this contract.

I had never signed a contract at my last place of employment, only a sign-on bonus in which they actually *gave* me money throughout the first two years that I worked for them. I was never required to pay back any amount of money if I left early. Also, since I wasn't technically a new graduate, already having had two years under my belt, I felt like I shouldn't be signing this. Instead of questioning it, I felt forced to sign because I had already moved and quit my other job, so I felt like I had no other choice. Plus, I figured I wasn't planning on being on this unit forever, just long enough to transfer to another unit. I tried to overlook this but then I also noticed that there were a total of seven new nurse hires for the Observation Unit at this orientation. Immediately I knew that this unit obviously had a low retention rate. My gut was telling me that I should've listened when I'd done a share day. But there was no turning back now.

Each of the new nurses were required to shadow another nurse on the unit for the next eight weeks until the educator and managers felt that we were capable of taking on patients on our own. Honestly, I didn't need this long of an orientation period because I had already done this at my previous job, which required much more skill. I really only needed to learn the hospital's and unit's policies, as well as the EMR system because it was different from what I was used to. However, due to the contract, I had no other choice.

It was about halfway through our orientation period when one night I came in to work, and one of the other new hires ended up having her own set of patients for this shift. I was a bit puzzled, as was she, because we were still technically supposed to be shadowing another nurse, which meant we weren't supposed to be in the "numbers" (lingo for census) just yet. Then, on another night, I had my own set of patients as well. Since this was starting to become a habit, I documented everything of course and spoke up to the unit educator about it. She agreed that this was not supposed to be happening and was unaware that it was even going on. I had a meeting with her and the assistant manager to discuss what was occurring. In this meeting, I expressed my concerns and stated that if they were not going to abide by the contract, then the contract should be null and void. The assistant manager got offended of course and tried to defend their actions, stating that they could take us off of orientation any time they wanted if they saw fit. However, there was no discussion nor anything in writing prior to this about releasing us, so how was that possible? Additionally, the educator agreed with the assistant manager, making me look stupid, like she hadn't just agreed with me prior to the meeting that this was wrong of them to be putting us by ourselves without notice. I was beyond livid at this point, but you always have to have a bigger plan. Little did they know, I had an idea brewing of my own.

I gathered up as much proof as possible. This included the contract we'd signed, each handwritten weekly schedule of the nurses scheduled to work, and the patient rooms assigned to them, etc. I emailed a couple different directors that might be able to assist me, but they redirected me to the director of nursing (DON). I also tried to get the other new hires on board to come with me when I went to meet with the DON, because power is in numbers. Of course, they all talked a good talk, but wouldn't back it up when it was time to do so. I understood that they were probably nervous to confront the issue and didn't want to do anything to jeopardize their jobs. Even though they weren't willing to fight the fight with me, I wasn't going to allow this to happen to me. I had had enough of the nurses bullying each other and management getting over on people. It's never-ending in the nursing field. Thankfully, the DON had replied to my email and was willing to meet with me. I had so many emotions because I didn't want this to get back to my nurse manager and that I'd be the talk of the unit. I didn't want me speaking up to cause me to lose my job; I didn't know whose side the DON would be on, a nurse manager or mine? Although retaliation is illegal, companies can always find a way around it.

I went in on my day off to meet with her. She greeted me and made me feel comfortable as I expressed to her how I felt and what exactly was going on. I showed her the documentation I had, and she was actually disgusted with what I was presenting to her. She couldn't believe this was happening, and she agreed with me that this was wrong. Additionally, she was going to discuss it further with my manager of course and make sure to type a formal letter stating that my contract was null and void. She said she'd email me a copy, as well as send a printed signed copy in the mail within the next 48 hours. Although the meeting went well, I still left there that day in fear of losing my job, not knowing if I could truly trust her. However, she kept her word, and I received an email within 24 hours with a letter stating my contract was null and void. I later received a signed copy of the letter in the mail.

I was so appreciative of her, but I still feared my managers would watch my every move just to try and find a way to get rid of me. With that said, that would never happen because I do not have a sloppy work ethic. I'm very punctual and consistent, and it shows in my work. I'm that Type A person that triple checks everything, especially when it comes to my job; I take that very seriously. Surprisingly, my managers never mentioned the letter or the meeting, and I wasn't going to say anything to them about it either. They actually asked me if I had any ideas of improving the unit and gave me a recognition certificate for doing a good job with a particular patient that was very pleased with me.

I was proud of myself for having the courage to do what was right and be my own advocate. Sometimes it's about principle, and that means speaking up for yourself and/or others. Don't ever think that your superiors are better than you or allow them to take advantage of a situation just because of their title, because they can be wrong also. After that situation and now being out of my contract, I knew it was time to be on the job hunt once again. I was no longer obligated to stay at this job. I began looking on multiple online job websites for open nursing positions that grabbed my interest.

21

Indeed For the Win

In the meantime, I still had my current job to tend to. As time went on, I began to notice that this was not a typical observation unit; this was basically another med-surg/tele unit. We admitted patients to the unit that really should've been sent to a more suitable unit. Observation meant a 24-48 hour stay, not a week or longer. We'd get patients that were on isolation precautions, which our unit was not equipped for since the rooms weren't designated negative pressure rooms with real doors, and there were only two bathrooms on the unit for 19 beds. That meant if a patient had Clostridium difficile (C-diff), everyone else was at risk of getting it because they'd be using the same bathroom. Unfortunately, the nurse director was in charge of both the emergency room (ER) and the observation unit. That meant that we really didn't have a say, especially since she had greater preference over the needs of the ER than the observation unit.

Since our nurse manager oversaw both the observation unit and the ER, that meant that if the ER was short and if the observation unit had a low census, one of the observation unit nurses would have to float to the ER to assist them. If the census started to pick up on our unit throughout the shift, then of course we'd be sent back to our unit to assist. None of the ER nurses ever floated to our floor even during the many times that we were trying to keep our head above water. I floated to the ER many times, and although I always felt a little anxious when it was my turn, it was definitely a good experience to have. The ER environment is much more fast-paced; you never know who or what kind of situation you're going to get. That's what makes it so fascinating and keeps you on your toes.

Some of the tasks that I did to assist the ER staff was starting an IV line, drawing STAT lab work, taking vitals, transferring a patient to another floor, and helping in a code or an emergency situation. The ER had been one of my interests at one point since the real life television show grasped my interest in the medical field in the first place. The ER wasn't the only floor I floated to while working at this hospital, as well as my previous employer. I had also floated to the Acute Care/Intermediate Care Unit (IMC), Acute Care/Cardiac Unit, Orthopedic Unit, and other Medical-Surgical/Telemetry units.

When you're floated to another unit, be prepared to get whatever patients the regularly staffed nurses don't want (trust me, it happens). Fortunately, I wasn't always given the short end of the stick, and some of the other staff were quite helpful while I spent my shift on their unit. Nursing is universal, so a nurse must always be prepared when their time comes to be floated to another floor. As long as you know your basic nursing skills, you'll be just fine.

Once again, I was being forced to do something that was not discussed with me beforehand. I came in one night for my shift and found out that I had been chosen to be the charge nurse for the night. I told the day shift charge nurse that I wasn't doing it because I had never been trained nor even had a discussion about it. It was only me and three of the nurses that were hired with me that were scheduled to work that night, and I was the one with the most hospital experience. The day shift charge nurse called the assistant nurse manager to clarify who should be charge nurse for the night. One of the other nurses scheduled that night agreed to be the charge nurse.

It wasn't that I couldn't do it, because I could have and ultimately had to do it eventually anyway. It was that yet again, I was being forced into something without clear communication or regard for the safety of the unit. This incident amongst all the others were the very reasons why I continued my job search even while having a job. It would motivate me to apply to as many jobs as I qualified for.

While looking outside of my current hospital, I was also inquiring about the Mother/Baby and NICU unit at my hospital. Unfortunately, the mother/baby nurse manager didn't agree to meet with me but told me if I had any questions that she could answer them via email. The NICU nurse manager responded back to my email, asking if I would like to do a four-hour shadow day. I agreed, and I truly enjoyed it; being there for those short four hours made me have much more respect for those nurses. It is amazing how well they take care of those little babies. They are so fragile, and it definitely takes a special person to work on that type of unit. It can be a very emotional environment. You're not just caring for the baby, you're also giving compassion for the parents as well.

I spoke to the nurse manager afterwards, which gave me a chance to express how much I wanted a change and for her to match my name to my face. She encouraged me to apply and said that she had a couple open positions. The only downside was yet another two-year commitment, rotating shifts, with a requirement to work four weekend days every four weeks. However, I still applied. I had to notify my current manager that I was putting in the application because they still had to approve the transfer if I got offered the position. Ultimately, I did not get the position. Although it very well could've been that the NICU manager chose the other candidates, I personally feel like my current manager blocked my transfer.

Knowing that it would be a difficult task to transfer to another unit within my hospital, I knew it was time to find employment elsewhere. I still wanted to do clinical work, but I wasn't sure if I wanted to be in a hospital setting. So I was looking for jobs in an office setting, hoping to have more of a structured schedule—all weekends/holidays off and no more night shifts. However, I knew that meant possibly taking a pay cut and of course not getting that differential pay. I began working with a nursing agency, and my recruiter sent me on several interviews. I also applied to jobs that I was interested in that I saw online. There was one job that I really wanted because it still allowed me to work with children, something I've always wanted to do. It was at a pediatric doctor's office, literally seven minutes from where I was living. After two interviews, I got the job! As excited as I was, I would've had to take a $5 pay cut, and they weren't willing to increase my pay at all. As much as I wanted the job, I couldn't afford to take such a pay cut, so I had to regretfully decline.

As I was still on the job search, an operating room (OR) position was presented to me by another recruiter from a different nursing agency. I was reluctant because it was yet another hospital with a stipulation of a two-year commitment and pay back penalty if I left before those two years were completed. I tried to be positive because I've always been interested in watching surgeries, and it could be a great experience. However, I had a friend from nursing school who had been working in the OR since we graduated, and I remember all her horror stories. She would tell me how rude and disrespectful the surgeons or senior staff were to her, and that's something I do not have the tolerance for. I had already dealt with that with seasoned nurses, and I didn't want to deal with that again with a surgeon. Taking a chance yet again, I went on the interview and accepted the job offer when notified that they wanted to hire me. This position was also a pay cut, but only $1, which I could work with, but no differential pay because I was working day shift. The payback penalty this time was $7500.

22

The Grass is STILL NOT Greener

The OR program consisted of six new hire nurses and we had to do classroom work (like we were in school) and ultimately get our experience shadowing another nurse/staff (circulator or scrub) during a surgery. We were supposed to (yeah, *SUPPOSED* to) have nine months of shadowing someone prior to being on our own and choosing what specialty we wanted to work in. Some of the different specialties consisted of robotics, plastics, cardiothoracic, gynecology & obstetrics, general, orthopedic, neurosurgery, oral & maxillofacial, colon & rectal, trauma, etc. Initially, the educators, lead RNs, and other staff were welcoming and willing to guide us; some of course were not. After about the first week, the other five nurses and I felt uneasy working there but did our best to stay positive since it was still early in the program. Apparently, that particular OR hires six new nurses every few months to do this program, and their retention rate is low. This became apparent as the days went on and we understood why.

The educators and most of the staff had negative attitudes and were not so helpful. Our preceptors started to leave us in a case without support after about two weeks of us working in the operating room, getting too comfortable thinking we were fine without them being in there. The preceptors that were assigned to us weren't just the regular staff, but sometimes the travel nurses who barely knew the routine of this OR and the surgeons' preferences. The educators literally put us wherever they could. If my preceptor left me in the room alone during a case, that really made me frustrated because if I needed them, they weren't there. During surgery, everyone must be attentive because of the high risks involved. Seeing all these issues, on top of a plethora of other things, I knew I still had to be on the job hunt because I knew this was definitely not where I wanted to stay. What put the nail in the coffin for me was when I was humiliated and disrespected by a surgeon. This surgeon had a reputation of being rude, and I had been in on his surgeries before but as a circulator RN. A circulator RN documents everything about the surgery in the computer and gets any supplies needed during surgery that aren't already in the room. The scrub is the one passing the surgical instruments to the surgeon during surgery.

During this day, I was the scrub. The regular scrub that worked with this surgeon was on PTO, so I was with someone else. The regular scrub and that surgeon had a closer relationship, so the scrub put him in his place when he was acting out of hand. The particular scrub that I had to shadow this day was not that assertive and wasn't well known to this surgeon, so I knew already that this was not going to be fun.

When you pass a surgical instrument to the surgeon, it has to be passed a particular way so that the surgeon doesn't have to adjust it or look away from the surgical field. I guess I wasn't passing them to his liking, even though I thought I was doing just fine, and my preceptor thought so also. As I was passing him an instrument, the surgeon got frustrated and basically told me I wasn't passing the instruments to him correctly, and he smacked the back of my hand.

I told him, "Please don't ever do that or touch me again."

He continued with his rude comments and went back to what he was doing. When I get mad, it's difficult for me to hide it and I tear up, not because I'm sad or hurt, but because I'm so infuriated and that's just how my emotions come out. I could feel my eyes start to water, and my preceptor looked at me and asked if I wanted to take a break. I initially told him no because I didn't want the surgeon to think I was weak. After a few minutes, I still couldn't allow myself to calm down, and I didn't want my tears to drop on the surgical field, so I told my preceptor I was going to step out for a few minutes. I couldn't get out of there fast enough.

As soon as I got back to the locker room, the tears just started flowing. I was so frustrated and wanted to go home so badly. The circulator RN had followed me and tried to be positive. She told me to come back and that he wasn't normally like that, but I didn't want to hear anything she was saying. Word must've gotten back to one of the educators because she came into the locker room shortly after that to see if I was okay and told me to come talk to her when I got myself together. I went to her office and explained what happened and she said that particular surgeon did this a lot, and that she and the director would have a talk with him. They didn't want me to be discouraged because of this and did reprimand him, but of course I'm sure he'll still continue to behave this way. I witnessed several other surgeons being disrespectful to other staff during surgeries, and these were seasoned staff that had been doing this for years.

I was shadowing a circulator RN one day for a thyroidectomy case. The scrub had years of experience and she had been working as a travel scrub for a little while now. Every surgeon has their preference in how they like their surgeries handled. This includes the specific brands of the surgical supplies they like to use, the kind of surgical tools and equipment they like to use, and how they want the room set up. It could be the exact same surgery between two different surgeons, but one likes their setup one way as opposed to another way. It could even be the same surgeon doing the same exact surgery on two different patients, but they may do one surgery differently than the other. This makes it difficult to have everything set up the correct way every time because things always change. Some surgeons are a bit more relaxed than others and don't let such miniscule aspects ruin the mood of the room.

This particular surgeon was a female, and she got upset twice with the scrub tech. It had something to do with the particular brand of surgical supplies that were available on the surgical tray. Usually there are note cards for each surgery that each surgeon does. It's supposed to be a reference so that the staff knows what supplies and equipment to have in the room for a particular surgery. These cards were also usually incorrect and not updated, so it was almost pointless to even follow them. That was simply what the staff went by for that surgery because the scrub, not the circulator, had been familiar with this particular surgeon. When the surgeon didn't like what was on the surgical tray, she yelled at the scrub and disrespected her in front of everyone else in the room. I felt so bad for her, but in that moment, who was I to speak up to that surgeon in defense of the scrub? That's how you feel when you witness something like that and you are still learning your way around a new environment.

I just think this type of culture is so disrespectful and counterproductive. If there is an issue, speak with the person privately after the surgery is over; don't humiliate them in front of everyone else. The patient on the operating table is most important, and everyone arguing at each other during this time is careless and unsafe. There is a way to correct someone professionally without all of the humiliating comments. This is why I knew I had to get out of that job as quickly as I could. Some say you have to have tough skin to work in the OR. To me, it's not about having tough skin; it's about having self-respect. I have too much respect for myself to allow someone to speak to me in that manner and humiliate me.

I explained my concerns to the recruiter who set me up for this job, and he was not very helpful at all, trying to convince me to stay at a place where I was unhappy. I didn't feel like he was on my side, and why would he be? He was probably getting paid from me staying at the job as long as possible. So the other recruiter from the other agency was finding me jobs that I was interested in, and I'd go on interviews, but nothing panned out. In the meantime, nurses that got hired in the group before us were leaving for the same reasons I wanted to leave. One of the other nurses hired at the same time left also. I was worried about having to pay the money back, but my happiness and sanity was so much more important. Plus, I'd find a loophole to get out of paying that money anyway.

23

Never Burn Your Bridges

hile on the job hunt, I was still in contact with my old preceptor/coworker TJ, whom I had worked with on the psych unit. She's always been like a big sister/mentor to me, always checking in on me no matter what. I've learned throughout the years to never burn your bridges because you never know when an opportunity can come your way. I was desperate at this point and as I was expressing my current situation to TJ, she told me there was an opening in her department. I knew if she loved this job then I would too. She told me all the perks, and I knew I had to give it a try. Although it didn't seem as exciting and fast-paced as I was used to, it seemed like a job that I could transition smoothly into.

Thankfully, she put in a good word for me and got me set up for an interview. I remember having that interview and another interview at a surgical center that day. The other interview was set up for me by the nursing recruiter that I had been working with. My first interview was with the insurance agency that TJ had set up for me, and it went very well. It was a panel interview with three different employees. I could tell they really liked me by the way they responded to my answers, and the HR representative basically told me they'd notify me of my second interview. I'd been told this before, and even though TJ put in a good word for me, I knew there were other candidates. I didn't want to get my hopes up, so I still proceeded with my interview at the surgical center. I didn't want to miss out on another opportunity if the first one didn't work out.

That interview went well also, but I knew that wasn't the job that I really wanted, and I didn't want to just settle because I wanted to leave my current job so badly. I've had these gut feelings before, yet I still gave them chances only to be unhappy and unfulfilled with the choice that I made. I was sure I could do the job, but my hours weren't a guaranteed 9-5 pm, and I'd have to get there early to set up for the day and couldn't leave until the last patient left. Once again, that meant having an unpredictable schedule and working longer hours than I intended to. Additionally, this job was 30 minutes from home, not including traffic.

The recruiter said that they really liked me, and she asked if I wanted her to push for me to get the position. I reluctantly told her no because I really wanted the job with the insurance agency. I didn't want to say yes to the surgical center and then turn around and tell them I couldn't do it because I'd chosen another job. I know most people would just say yes to an offer so that they at least had something to fall back on, because I'm sure the surgical center had other prospects. However, they might not have, and I didn't want to hold up their hiring process knowing that I really didn't want to be there anyway.

So I waited patiently to hear back from the insurance agency. They contacted me and I had my second interview with the manager. This was more personable because it was just me and her; I felt more relaxed but still nervous as I usually am in interviews, as many times as I've been on them. She loved me and told me she couldn't wait for me to start. I was so excited and thankful for this opportunity. I was also nervous that I'd become bored because I'd be on a computer all day with no more clinical/hands-on experience. However, I knew that if TJ had so many positive things to say about this job, then I would definitely enjoy working there. The icing on the cake was the fact that my job offer included a salary higher than I'd requested. It has been quite a challenge getting pay increases from the beginning of my journey, so I was truly honored to receive this offer.

It was now time to quit my job in the OR. I had only been there for four months, the shortest nursing job that I'd had thus far. I worried about having to pay back that money for not fulfilling my time, but I knew that my happiness and sanity meant so much more. I had student loans I was still paying for, so this wouldn't be any different; they'd get what I could give and not a penny more. Plus, I truly felt that that was just a ploy to scare new hires to stay, especially with that outrageous amount they expected you to pay back; I was willing to take my chances. Some of the nurses hired for the OR transferred to the pre-operative floor, Post-Anesthesia Care Unit (PACU), or a med-surg/tele unit in the same hospital just so they wouldn't have to pay back the money. I just couldn't see myself on another hospital floor and definitely not at that hospital.

Thanksgiving was approaching, and I was going to have that Thursday (Thanksgiving day) and I had taken Black Friday off also. So I sent my resignation to the OR director, who I'd interviewed with, that Black Friday. I made sure to carbon coby (CC) another faculty member as well, so that my words would not be misconstrued. I basically expressed how I felt about the program and the other staff I'd encountered, how much disrespect I had not only observed but personally experienced as well. Even if they never sought to improve the culture of their OR, I at least felt like I should express my experience because I knew of so many other nurses who either left or wanted to leave but didn't and who felt the same way I did. I never got a response from her, of course. I received a text from one of the clinical educators that following week asking me to return the books they had loaned to us for our classroom assignments. Thankfully, one of the other nurses in my group agreed to return them for me since I had purposely left them in my work locker so that I didn't have to ever go back there again. The fact that they didn't feel the need to provide any feedback from my email just shows me that I made the right decision to leave.

I still received my last paycheck plus an extra paycheck for my unused PTO. I also received a letter in the mail almost three months later from the hospital's HR department basically telling me I needed to pay back the $7500 within a month or their legal department would step in. Honestly, that scare tactic didn't work. I simply responded to the letter in an email addressed to the HR representative, expressing how I don't feel like I owed any money back due to the fact that the program didn't hold up their side of the deal. I also discussed their constant turnover rate, lack of professionalism, and proof and witnesses that I had of all these instances. Once again, I never heard anything back, and that was February of 2017. One of the other nurses that left before me told me she received the same letter and responded similarly as well. She never heard anything back after she responded either.

I will never allow anyone to bully me into anything, especially when it comes to a profession that I worked so hard to get into. I will always stand up for what I believe in and always stay true to myself. That being said, I knew that I had made the right decision leaving that job and coming to work for the insurance agency. There was no turning back now; I was now off to my office job where I could still use all that I had learned and experienced. Little did I know then how much those experiences would help in my current job.

24

Final Destination

*I*t was the start of my new job, and I was already enjoying having my own cubicle. I can honestly say that it was a struggle to stay focused in the beginning because it had been so long since I'd had a desk job. I hadn't had a desk job since college, so it took some getting used to the slow-paced environment again. I was used to the constant hustle and bustle of working on the floor in the hospital, with little to no breaks. So to sit down and do my work at my own pace within a quiet environment was a whole new experience for me. Additionally, training with someone and mostly having to watch how to do the work before you're able to do it on your own can drag the workday out longer.

It didn't take me long to pick up on the work since I am a fast learner and know my way around a computer. I had two nurses training me on opposite weeks; they both had different learning styles which were beneficial for me in the grand scheme of things. Once the two nurses training me felt that I understood the basics, they allowed me some more independence. I would do my work and they would check to make sure I had the correct responses. This in-office training went on for the first six months of working there. After that, I had the opportunity to start working from home, but I was still required to come into the office once a week and for mandatory meetings.

I was thrilled because this meant not having to wake up early to beat the traffic, not having to get dressed up, not having to pack my breakfast/lunch, saving gas, and the flexibility of it all. Additionally, I received four weeks of PTO, a raise and bonus every year, great medical benefits, and other perks. Now I personally knew why TJ loved this job so much!

Although I am no longer doing in-person patient care, I am still utilizing my knowledge and skill to still provide the best care possible for those policy holders and their families. I still oversee their visits/surgeries through reviewing their claims and medical records. I can honestly say that I enjoy my job and couldn't see myself anywhere else at this point in my life. With being a first-time mom, I couldn't ask for a better job. It allows more flexibility and a better work/home life balance. Of course, I still deal with coworkers who may smile in my face but talk about me behind my back, but that's going to happen at any job. As long as I know I'm doing my job well and my supervisor and manager constantly appreciate the work that I do, that's all that matters to me. I probably am more appreciated at this job than any other job that I've had as a nurse. It definitely boosts my confidence and makes me feel needed and not just easily replaceable. They really do have my best interests at heart.

I do plan to move up the totem pole within this company the more I learn and gain more confidence with the work that I do. I got a senior nurse promotion in the second year of working there. That tells me that my work does not go unnoticed. I can't tell you what the future holds for me, but I know that it will be positive. My path may not be your path, but that is why there is a job out there for every individual. What I may be able to handle another person may not, and vice versa. I say this to encourage you to find your path in nursing. Know that no experience should be a regret or taken for granted because all of those experiences mold us into who we are today, the good and the bad.

I say this to emphasize that nursing is so broad, with a plethora of job opportunities. One does not need to settle on one particular setting. A lot of people may think the only setting for a nurse is "in the hospital," but that is far from true. Of course you'll get more hands-on clinical experience by working in the hospital, having X amount of patients to care for on a particular shift, but nursing has so much more to offer. As I've shared with you, within those first three years of being a nurse, I worked on four different units in three different hospitals. While being a CNA in nursing school, I did home health and worked in a separate hospital from the three that I was working as a nurse in. I also was a flu nurse during one flu season, giving out flu shots to the public. Now I'm currently working in health insurance.

If you had asked me five years ago where I saw myself working, I would've never guessed that I'd be where I am currently. I had a much different desire and outlook on what that would be. Honestly, I thought I'd get bored with this job and that it wouldn't be as fast paced as I needed it to be. However, the way that my life is right now makes this the best position that I could be in. I had several former colleagues and nursing friends inquire about my current job the moment I started. Just about all of them have families, including young children. They were looking for a job with a better, more flexible schedule to give them a better work/home life balance. They knew that's what I currently have, and that's what they're yearning for. I am happy to guide them in the right direction so that they can seek a similar position that meets their needs.

I'm also a member of a social media nursing group, and several of them have questioned their career as well. They wonder if this is truly their calling, or if they should quit. Depending on the demand of their job, in any field actually, can truly make you question the choice that you made. However, it may not be that you are in the wrong career; it just may be that your current job is wrong for you. I can definitely say that before I acquired this position, I did not love my job. I'd wanted to be a nurse for so long, and I started hating it; I was becoming overwhelmed. My blood pressure even started being elevated because of the stress. I knew that I couldn't settle for a job like this. As we know, everyone is replaceable, and that same job will hire someone else the very moment you either leave or expire. You have to truly find a job that cares about their employees or create that job for yourself.

It's all about finding the job you can truly fall in love with that will encourage you to stay on your path. You just have to find your niche. Nurses are needed as travel nurses, informatics, school nurses, home health nurses, correctional nurses, nurse practitioners, DNPs, surgery center nurses, health insurance, etc. This field is not limited, and that means that you don't have to limit what you choose to do in this field. Test the waters and find the right fit for you. That's what I did. Life changes, and your interests change, so do what makes you happy. In the end, that's what truly matters.

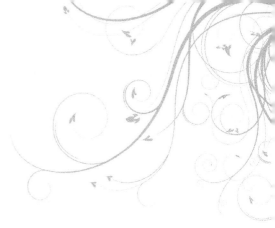

Conclusion

$\mathcal{A}$ lthough my journey as a registered nurse may not be labeled as "seasoned" to most, I feel as though I have experienced plenty of aspects of nursing in my seven years. This journey has given me a voice to speak out to other potential nurses, or those who are already in the field, even those that may have been in the game longer than I have. We can all learn from each other's stories, no matter how old or young, new or seasoned; everyone has their own experience. This book isn't meant for you to follow my exact footsteps, but it is to give you a short blueprint on what to expect.

No matter how we managed to get to becoming a nurse, we all experience similar aspects of this job. Nursing can definitely be a challenging job, but it has so many rewards that you would never imagine. A nurse gets to be someone's saving grace, a shoulder to cry on, that one person that a patient can count on to show up. I've seen patients that didn't have family or a good support system, and they yearn for that attention. You may think that they're holding you up from getting to the next patient or they may seem like they're "nagging" you, but in reality, you may be all that person has to look forward to every day. That in itself is a blessing, because something so small to you means the world to them.

Nursing is about compassion, patience, and empathy. Ask yourself, do you have all of those qualities? These qualities are so important when entering this field. If one day, you realize those qualities don't exist for you anymore, truly question if this field is still the right fit for you. Remember that there are so many different areas of nursing offered to us, you don't need to settle on one area. Your current position just may have run its course. I know my position in the hospital did, and thankfully I am where I am meant to be in this part of my life.

Although I could never see myself working in a hospital environment again, especially with the high risks of Covid-19, I truly am glad that I got the experience that I did. I salute all my fellow healthcare workers for dedicating themselves during these uncertain times, as well as all essential personnel. Those experiences have shaped me into the person that I am today, both professionally and personally. Always stand up for yourself and be confident, because this career field is truly not for the weak. Remember why you chose this profession and when you think of giving up, think of that reason to pick yourself back up. I hope that this book finds you well and wish you all the best in your future or current endeavors. Always remember........DOCUMENT DOCUMENT DOCUMENT.

Acknowledgements

*E*veryone has a story to tell, but I never thought that my story was inspiring enough. I am forever grateful for my partner and the father of our child, Cliff, for always pushing me to finish this book from day one. He believed in me, and in turn, I believed in myself.

I also appreciate the many talks with one of my closest friends, Shardae, for keeping my eyes on the prize. We started this nursing journey together, and I am honored to still have her in my life.

Last but not least, I am truly thankful for *13th and Joan Publishing House*. They believed in my story and took a chance on me. Without them, this book wouldn't be all that it has to offer.

About the Author

*D*eanna Mackey is a registered nurse with experience in several areas of nursing. Her experience in these different areas of nursing has allowed her to understand nursing and healthcare on a deeper level. She believes that her personal accounts should be shared to spread knowledge to answer questions inquiring minds want to know and to know what to expect when you choose to be a part of this field. She is passionate about health and has recently started juicing in her spare time to assist those interested in gaining a healthier lifestyle.

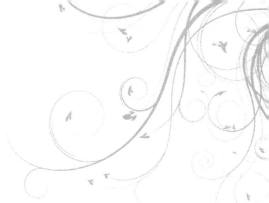

Get Connected

Instagram:	queenofhealthdeanna (personal)
	raine_n_juice (juicing page)
Twitter:	queenofhealthdm
Facebook fanpage:	queenofhealthdeanna
Juicing Facebook page:	Raine'N Juice
LinkedIn:	Deanna Mackey
Email:	queenofhealthdeanna@gmail.com
Website:	https://queenofhealthdeanna.com